# MEDICAL QUALITY MANAGEMENT

## THEORY AND PRACTICE

D1368305

American College of Medical Quality
*Editor: Prathibha Varkey*

**JONES AND BARTLETT PUBLISHERS**

*Sudbury, Massachusetts*

BOSTON    TORONTO    LONDON    SINGAPORE

## World Headquarters

Jones and Bartlett Publishers
40 Tall Pine Drive
Sudbury, MA 01776
978-443-5000
info@jbpub.com
www.jbpub.com

Jones and Bartlett Publishers
Canada
6339 Ormindale Way
Mississauga, Ontario L5V 1J2
Canada

Jones and Bartlett Publishers
International
Barb House, Barb Mews
London W6 7PA
United Kingdom

Jones and Bartlett's books and products are available through most bookstores and online booksellers. To contact Jones and Bartlett Publishers directly, call 800-832-0034, fax 978-443-8000, or visit our website www.jbpub.com.

Substantial discounts on bulk quantities of Jones and Bartlett's publications are available to corporations, professional associations, and other qualified organizations. For details and specific discount information, contact the special sales department at Jones and Bartlett via the above contact information or send an email to specialsales@jbpub.com.

The authors, editor, and publisher have made every effort to provide accurate information. However, they are not responsible for errors, omissions, or for any outcomes related to the use of the contents of this book and take no responsibility for the use of the products and procedures described. Treatments and side effects described in this book may not be applicable to all people; likewise, some people may require a dose or experience a side effect that is not described herein. Drugs and medical devices are discussed that may have limited availability controlled by the Food and Drug Administration (FDA) for use only in a research study or clinical trial. Research, clinical practice, and government regulations often change the accepted standard in this field. When consideration is being given to use of any drug in the clinical setting, the health care provider or reader is responsible for determining FDA status of the drug, reading the package insert, and reviewing prescribing information for the most up-to-date recommendations on dose, precautions, and contraindications, and determining the appropriate usage for the product. This is especially important in the case of drugs that are new or seldom used.

### Production Credits

Publisher: David Cella
Associate Editor: Maro Gartside
Production Manager: Julie Champagne Bolduc
Production Assistant: Jessica Steele Newfell
Senior Marketing Manager: Barb Bartoszek
Associate Marketing Manager: Lisa Gordon
Manufacturing and Inventory Control Supervisor:
  Amy Bacus
Composition: Spearhead, Inc.
Cover Design: Timothy Dziewit
Printing and Binding: Malloy, Inc.
Cover Printing: Malloy, Inc.

### Library of Congress Cataloging-in-Publication Data

Medical quality management : theory and practice / American College of Medical Quality. — 2nd ed.
  p. ; cm.
  Rev. ed. of: Core curriculum for medical quality management/American College of Medical Quality c2005.
  Includes bibliographical references and index.
  ISBN 978-0-7637-6034-2 (pbk. : alk. paper)
1. Medical care—United States—Quality control—Outlines, syllabi, etc. 2. Total quality management—United States—Outlines, syllabi, etc. I. American College of Medical Quality. II. Core curriculum for medical quality.
  [DNLM: 1. Quality of Health Care—organization & administration. W 84.1 M4896 2009]
  RA399.A3C667 2010
  362.1068—dc22

                2008048845

6048

Printed in the United States of America
13  12  11  10  09    10  9  8  7  6  5  4  3  2  1

# Contents

## Chapter 2   Quality Measurement    29

**Linda Harrington, PhD, RN, CNS, CPHQ, *and***
**Harry Pigman, MD, MSHP**

| **Chapter 3** | **Patient Safety** | **43** |
|---|---|---|

*Philip J. Fracica, MD, MBA, FACP, Sharon Wilson, RN, BS, PMP, and Lakshmi P. Chelluri, MD, MPH, CMQ*

**Chapter 4 Organization Design and Management**     **75**

**James T. Ziegenfuss, Jr., PhD, and
Thomas Biancaniello, MD, FACC**

## Chapter 5  Medical Informatics                                    89

*Louis H. Diamond, MB, ChB, FACP, and*
*Stephen T. Lawless, MD, MBA*

## Chapter 6 Economics and Finance in Medical Quality Management 111

*Donald Fetterolf, MD, MBA, FACP, and*
*Rahul K. Shah, MD, FAAP*

## Chapter 7  Utilization Management — 145
*Arthur L. Pelberg, MD, MPA*

## Chapter 8  External Quality Improvement: Accreditation, Quality Improvement Education, and Certification    167
*Toni Kfuri, MD, MPH, CMQ, FACOG, and Nancy L. Davis, PhD*

## Chapter 9  Interfaces Between Quality Improvement, Law, and Medical Ethics    197
*Jeffrey M. Zale, MD, MPH, CMQ, and Mano S. Selvan, PhD*

# Foreword

*Carolyn M. Clancy, MD*

*Director, Agency for Healthcare Research and Quality (AHRQ)*

*Education is the most powerful weapon which you can use to change the world.*
— *Nelson Mandela*

*They say that time changes things, but you actually have to change them yourself.*
— *Andy Warhol*

Only four years have passed since the book *Core Curriculum for Medical Quality Management* was published in 2005. Since then, the field of quality improvement has seen major progress in the impact of its research findings, the adoption of technology to promote safety and enhance quality, and the dissemination of clinical and organizational case studies.

Against this backdrop, the American College of Medical Quality has wisely decided to issue this revised edition. As a physician and a director of a federal health research agency, I am gratified to see both the faster pace of progress on quality improvement and the commitment that this book makes to educate new and experienced health professionals.

Whether you have worked in quality improvement for 20 years or 20 days, I urge you to thoroughly educate yourself on patient safety, to which an extensive chapter in this book is devoted. As public and private sector policies evolve, the reputation, clinical excellence, and financial success of your organization will depend greatly on patient safety outcomes.

A timely chapter on medical informatics is a comprehensive resource on standards and data, state and national information systems, data sets and coding systems, and case studies. Research projects on health information technology funded by my agency continue to underscore both the challenges of implementation and the tremendous opportunities for improved safety and quality.

Topics that are the bread and butter of medical quality management—quality measurement, utilization management, accreditation, education, and certification—receive a thorough examination in this edition. They also benefit from the addition of new case studies, which provide a valuable "real-world" element and a look at future trends.

The American College of Medical Quality continues to be a national leader in educating the medical community about both the science and the practice of medical quality management. The new edition of this book underscores the College's commitment to our shared vision of a safer health care system and provides many resources to readers that will guide our journey.

# Introduction

*Alex R. Rodriguez, MD*

*Medical quality management* is a term that has yet to find its way into any leading compendium of health care definitions. Nevertheless, it represents an area in which almost all physicians in active clinical practice are engaged on a daily basis as well as the primary field of professional action for an estimated 16,000 physicians in the United States and an unknown but growing number internationally. Medical quality management (MQM) is elemental to clinical services and has been recognized as an area of medical specialization by the American Medical Association for 20 years, but public recognition of the field needs a strong boost.

While many health care professionals become engaged in MQM activities over the course of their clinical careers, only a few have received any formal training or orientation in the field during their undergraduate or postgraduate professional training. During their formative training, medical and nursing students and residents may become aware that some licensed professionals are involved in utilization review, quality improvement, and risk management activities; however, few are aware of the rich scientific base and health tradition that frames the field.

Dr. Avedis Donabedian initially termed the professional practice field *clinical outcomes management*, which was later popularized by Dr. Paul Ellwood's seminal 1988 Shattuck Lecture published in the *New England Journal of Medicine*.[1,2] Since then, only two major texts have provided summations of the essential components of MQM: *Health Care Quality Management for the 21st Century*, edited by James Couch, MD, JD, and *Core Curriculum for Medical Quality Management*, published by the American College of Medical Quality (ACMQ), the latter of which provides the most recent compendium of the elemental knowledge base for the field of MQM.[3,4]

*Medical Quality Management: Theory and Practice* has been written and edited as a basic text to describe the key components of MQM. As such, this text has applicability for novices, committed students, and seasoned practitioners within the field. Each chapter has been designed for a review of the essential history, precepts, and exemplary practices within the area of review. A common format is followed within the chapters to provide structure to the authors' comments, including useful learning objectives, case studies, interchapter cross-references, and substantial references. While no single chapter does, or could, provide a comprehensive or in-depth summation of the respective area, each reliably captures the essential elements that will allow a diligent reader to establish a practical fluency in the topic. The authors are all noted experts in their topical areas and have encapsulated their respective knowledge and experience bases into exceptionally well-researched and written summaries. Individual chapters focus on the following core curriculum essentials.

Varkey, in Chapter 1, sets the tone and foundation for the book by highlighting the basic historical drivers of medical quality assurance and quality improvement, by reviewing the major concepts and common applications of quality improvement (QI) methods and strategies and by outlining the challenges and opportunities within the rapidly evolving field of MQM. The chapter opens the door to a sometimes-complex field of quality measurement methods and systems, operational processes, and strategies.

In Chapter 2, Harrington and Pigman focus on the history, types, characteristics, processes, and interpretations of quality measurements. They provide a framework for understanding the basic components of quality measurement within direct care and policy-making settings, exemplified by illustrative case studies. They effectively correlate the critical interface of quality measurement strategies and methods to areas highlighted in other chapters, especially medical informatics, utilization and quality management, patient safety, and health policy development.

In Chapter 3, Fracica, Wilson, and Chelluri provide a detailed overview of the major patient safety concepts, medical error categories and causal factors, techniques and tools for systematic patient safety enhancement (PSE), and future trends. Particular attention is directed to the prevention of adverse drug events, invasive procedures, and common risk situations. They also focus on attributes of high-reliability organizations and operational interventions for PSE. The national momentum towards substantive investments in patient safety prevention, tracking, and educational systems represents a true megatrend in health care and a core area of focus in MQM.

Ziegenfuss and Biancaniello focus on organizational design and leadership in Chapter 4. Most of the publications in these areas tend to be theoretical and descriptive, rather than framed by the numbers and the facts with which most health professionals are familiar. The discussions on quality management leadership, collaboration, strategic and operational planning, implementation, data analysis, and feedback are all presented clearly and—like all of the chapters—with an abundance of relevant references.

Diamond and Lawless, in Chapter 5, address developments and challenges within medical informatics, a central component of MQM that is taking on a more important role in health care. The authors concretely summarize the major developments of medical informatics infrastructures, including clinical decision support systems and tools and systems for data coding, transmission, quality control, storage, and analysis. While many might decry the current state of medical informatics in the United States, it is reflective of the experimental phase that is evolving within diverse commercial and regulated environments. The ultimate movement towards a uniquely American system of health care in a regulated marketplace will require a complex system of medical informatics in order to realize Dr. Ellwood's imagined national system of outcomes management.[2]

In Chapter 6, Fetterolf and Shah present the subject of economics and finance in MQM with a detailed approach. They elaborate on major economic and business principles relevant to the future practice of MQM, including those related to accounting and finance, organizational planning and psychology, project management, the development of business plans and financial statements, and sensitivity analyses. MQM professionals will need to make the business case for clinical services, framed by quality management objectives and outcomes metrics. The authors elegantly frame the lessons in this chapter, including several instructive case studies.

Reflective of the history of ACMQ, Pelberg reviews the past, the present, and the future of health care utilization management (UM) in Chapter 7. This chapter describes the essential processes, tasks, and common systems of UM with a focus on prior authorization, concurrent, and retrospective forms of utilization review to establish "medical necessity" of care. Medical necessity criteria, processes for determining the effectiveness and value of UM procedures (e.g., over- and underutilization markers), common organizational structures for UM activities, and accreditation standards and programs are also detailed. New sections in this chapter include a discussion of the role of UM in disease management, pay-for-performance programs, and models of care. This section is particularly important due to the current focus on the coordination of care models to make improvements in cost and quality.

In Chapter 8, Kfuri and Davis focus on key external QI activities, including accreditation, education, and professional certification. They highlight major health care standards-setting and accreditation organizations, including medical specialty board certification, state professional licensing, and prominent national accreditation organizations such as the National Committee for Quality Assurance (NCQA), Utilization Review Accreditation Commission (URAC), and the Joint Commission (TJC). These organizations promote continuous quality improvement methods and offer consumers, purchasers, regulators, providers, and managed care organizations consensus sets of quality control standards for health care quality management functions. As such, they serve to integrate the diverse number of utilization, quality, and risk management activities that frame clinical systems of care. The chapter includes a new focus on the importance of QI education for medical students and practicing physicians.

Finally, Zale and Selvan review the basic concepts, social institutions, legal requirements, and prevailing values that affect quality in Chapter 9. The authors review several current major national legal mechanisms for quality promotion such as the National Practitioner Data Bank, accreditation activities, peer review protections, the tort system, clinical practice guidelines, institutional review boards, and medical ethics programs. The chapter also provides thoughtful commentary about evolving trends aimed at improving the quality of health care service and delivery. Notable current movements that are evolving include how to handle apologies when a medical error has occurred, patient safety activities, and pay-for-performance initiatives.

These diverse, but intertwined, chapters provide the foundation upon which the specialty of medical quality management is now practiced. When John Williamson wrote the first instructional text on quality assurance in 1982, he had no way of knowing how much the field he then described would change in the ensuing years.[5] It is clear that quality will be both an expected outcome and a currency in the marketplace in the future and that professional leadership—based on specialized training, credentials, and experiences in medical quality management—will be required.

This book provides a portal into the brave new world of health care, one that increasingly will look to medical quality management professionals for guidance and leadership. It is a world that will require collaboration among professionals from the diverse fields of clinical science, health law, government regulations, public health, information technology, business, and consumerism in order to best assure that quality, as variously defined, is reliably achieved. As you read through this book, you will be invited to enter into that domain as students and as practitioners of the specialty of MQM. Following that exploration, it is the fervent hope of ACMQ that you will be better prepared to become an active leader in the ultimate quest of all enlightened health care systems—to improve the length and the quality of life of all who seek health care services.

## References

1. Donabedian A. *A Position Paper on the Future of ACURP*. Ann Arbor: University of Michigan Press; 1986.
2. Ellwood PM. Outcomes management: a technology of patient experience. *NEJM*. 1988; 318:1549–1556.
3. Couch JB. *Health Care Quality Management for the 21st Century*. Tampa, FL: American College of Physician Executives; 1991.
4. American College of Medical Quality. *Core Curriculum for Medical Quality Management*. Sudbury, MA: Jones and Bartlett; 2005.
5. Williamson JW. *Teaching Quality Assurance and Cost Containment in Health Care*. San Francisco: Jossey-Bass; 1982.

# Contributors

## Project Editor and Author

**Prathibha Varkey, MD, MPH, MHPE**, Associate Professor of Preventive Medicine, of Internal Medicine, and of Medical Education at Mayo Clinic, Rochester, Minnesota, and Associate Chair of the Department of Medicine. She is also Program Director for the Preventive Medicine Fellowship at Mayo and the Director of Quality at the Division of Preventive and Occupational Medicine at Mayo Clinic. Until recently she was the Director of Quality at Mayo School of Graduate Medical Education and Mayo School of Continuing Medical Education.

## Authors

**Thomas Biancaniello, MD, FACC**, Professor of Pediatrics and Medicine at the School of Medicine at Stony Brook University and Chief of the Division of Pediatric Cardiology. He also is Vice Dean for Clinical Affairs at the School of Medicine and Chief Medical Officer of Stony Brook University Hospital.

**Lakshmi P. Chelluri, MD, MPH, CMQ**, Professor in the Department of Critical Care Medicine, University of Pittsburgh School of Medicine, Co-Medical Director for Respiratory Care at UPMC Presbyterian, and Co-Medical Director for Critical Care Outreach, UPMC Presbyterian, Pittsburgh, Pennsylvania. Dr. Chelluri coordinates a curriculum in quality improvement–patient safety activities for adult critical care trainees.

**Nancy L. Davis, PhD**, Executive Director, National Institute for Quality Improvement and Education, a nonprofit organization dedicated to the integration of quality improvement and continuing medical education. She currently serves as the Chair of CME for the American College of Medical Quality, is past president of the Society for Academic CME, and is past chair of the Council of Medical Specialty Societies CME Directors' Group.

**Louis H. Diamond, MB, ChB, FACP**, Vice President and Medical Director at Thomson Reuters. He currently serves as President of the American College of Medical Quality, Chair of the Planning Advisory Committee for the Physician Consortium for Performance Improvement, President of the End-Stage Renal Disease Network 5, and Chair of the Quality Measurement, Research and Improvement Council for the National Quality Forum. He was previously Chairman of the Georgetown Department of Medicine at D.C. General Hospital and Professor of Medicine and Associate Dean for Medical Affairs at Georgetown School of Medicine.

**Donald Fetterolf, MD, MBA, FACP**, Executive Vice President, Health Intelligence at Matria Healthcare, Inc., a disease management organization based in Atlanta with operations throughout the United States. He is on the editorial board of several journals, including *Disease Management* and the *American Journal of Medical Quality*.

**Philip J. Fracica, MD, MBA, FACP**, Hospital Medical Director for Heartland Regional Medical Center in St. Joseph, Missouri. He serves as Medical Director for Case Management and as Chair of the Quality Management Board. He also serves as the Northwest Missouri Regional Medical Director for the Missouri Area Health Education Centers (MAHEC) program and is a past Medical Director for Donor Network of Arizona.

**Linda Harrington, PhD, RN, CNS, CPHQ**, Vice President for Advanced Nursing Practice at Baylor Health Care System, where she is responsible for nursing quality and research. Dr. Harrington also is an Adjunct Professor at Texas Christian University where she teaches population statistics and process statistics used in quality improvement.

**Toni E. Kfuri, MD, MPH, CMQ, FACOG**, Research Scientist at the Johns Hopkins School of Public Health, Department of Health, Policy and Management, with a focus on the development of clinical performance indicators in health informatics. He is a senior member and lead judge for the American Society for Quality and a national examiner in health care for the Malcolm Baldrige National Quality Awards program.

**Stephen T. Lawless, MD, MBA**, Vice President of Quality and Safety for Nemours, with responsibility for the oversight and coordination of quality and safety within all of Nemours. He is a Professor of Pediatrics at Thomas Jefferson University and Staff Intensivist in the Department of Anesthesiology and Critical Care Medicine at Alfred I. duPont Hospital for Children in Wilmington, Delaware.

**Arthur L. Pelberg, MD, MPA**, President of the Pelberg Group, a health care consulting group in quality, utilization, and physician mentoring. Dr. Pelberg serves in an advisory capacity to INSPIRUS of Arizona, a health care management company focused on improving care for the frail and elderly populations. He is past President and Chief Medical

Officer of Schaller Anderson, Inc. in Phoenix, Arizona, a health care management and consulting firm with operations across the United States.

**Harry Pigman, MD, MSPH**, Clinical Director of the South Central Veterans Health Care Network Data Warehouse. He currently oversees the use of a data repository for tracking processes and outcomes in a network of 10 VA medical centers. He has led both the Informatics Council and Quality Council for his network as well as several national quality efforts in the VA system, including the redesign of the ambulatory information system and the implementation of advanced clinical access.

**Alex R. Rodriguez, MD**, Chief Clinical Officer and Medical Director for Harmony Behavioral Health (WellCare Health Plans). He previously served as Chief Medical Officer for three national managed care organizations (Consortium Health Plans, Magellan Health Services, Preferred Health Care) and at CHAMPUS (Department of Defense). Prior to those assignments, he served as Special Assistant to two Secretaries of the U.S. Department of Health and Human Services and was a White House Fellow.

**Mano S. Selvan, PhD**, Health Care Researcher and Statistician in the Information Systems Division, Memorial Hermann Hospital, Houston, Texas. She has a PhD in social psychology from Bharathiar University in India and a master's degree in biostatistics from the University of Texas School of Public Health.

**Rahul K. Shah, MD, FAAP**, Assistant Professor of Otolaryngology and Pediatrics at Children's National Medical Center and George Washington University Medical Center, Washington, DC. Dr. Shah is an active clinical researcher, has received numerous awards for his research and is recognized as a leader in patient safety and quality improvement in the specialty of otolaryngology.

**Sharon Wilson, RN, BS, PMP**, Director of Idaho Medicare Operations at Qualis Health, the Quality Improvement Organization for Idaho and Washington. Her background includes executive director and senior management-level work in hospitals, managed care, and nonprofit settings. She has a BS degree in health care management. Ms. Wilson is certified as a Project Management Professional and is a Patient Safety Improvement Corp graduate.

**Jeffrey M. Zale, MD, MPH, CMQ**, Medical Director at the Delmarva Foundation, the Maryland and District of Columbia Quality Improvement Organization, with responsibilities including quality assurance, quality improvement, peer review, and external quality review for Medicaid managed care organizations.

**James T. Ziegenfuss, Jr., PhD**, Professor of Management and Health Care Systems in the Graduate Programs in Health and Public Administration, School of Public Affairs, Pennsylvania State University, where he is Adjunct Professor of Medicine. He was founding coordinator of the graduate program in health administration and teaches courses in strategic planning, health systems, quality management, organization behavior, and organization management consulting.

# Chapter 1

# Basics of Quality Improvement

*Prathibha Varkey, MD, MPH, MHPE*

## Executive Summary

The improvement in patient outcomes has been the primary objective of quality management practitioners since the publication of Codman's work nearly 100 years ago.[1] In this vein, the Institute of Medicine (IOM) defines *quality of care* as the degree to which health services increase the likelihood of desired health outcomes and are consistent with current professional knowledge. The Agency for Healthcare Research and Quality (AHRQ) describes quality improvement (QI) as "doing the right thing at the right time for the right individual to get the best possible results."[2] With the increasing focus on medical errors, cost-effective medicine, public reporting, and pay-for-performance, physicians, payers, and patients have turned to QI as a strategy and framework to address some of the concerns with the current health care system. Crosby suggests that poor quality not only affects patients negatively, but it also squanders resources that could be used to treat other patients.[3] Internal QI is vital to the ability of a health care organization or a practice to fulfill the fiduciary relationship between the physician and the patient; enhance medical care and care delivery; simplify and streamline procedures; reduce costs; increase patient and provider satisfaction; and enhance workplace morale and productivity. External QI is crucial for physician education, physician licensure and certification, benchmarking, accreditation, and health policy formulation.

This chapter introduces quality management theories and practices that have evolved over the past 25 years and highlights some of the themes that have marked the progress of the field. It also addresses points of philosophy and practice that characterize the QI field today.

## Learning Objectives

Upon completion of this chapter, readers should be able to:

- describe the history of QI in the field of health care;
- describe the purpose and philosophy of QI;
- describe the tools, methods, and strategies for successful QI in health care; and
- list the key evidence-based QI initiatives that affect patient outcomes.

## The History of the Health Care Quality Management Movement: Past to Present

In 1914, a surgeon named Ernest Codman developed one of the earliest initiatives in health care quality and challenged hospitals and physicians to take responsibility for the outcomes of their patients.[1] He called for a compilation and analysis of surgical outcomes. He recorded pertinent data (patient case numbers, preoperative diagnoses, members of the operating team, procedures, and results) on pocket-sized cards, which he then used to study outcomes.

Following Codman's early efforts, the next 6 to 7 decades focused primarily on evaluating poor outcomes and departures from standards, commonly referred to as *quality assurance* or *quality control*. This method focused on identifying deficient practitioners and mandating "improvements" (e.g., negative incentives, weeding out recalcitrant clinicians who refused to change). This narrow focus did not acknowledge the contribution of other organizational characteristics to QI, such as leadership, resources, information systems, communication patterns among teams, or the patient's perception of quality.

In the 1960s, Avedis Donabedian created the structure, the process, and the outcome paradigm for assessing quality in health care[4] that had such a profound influence that he is often thought of as the modern founder and leader of the quality field. His work influenced practitioners to identify various methods to enhance patient outcomes in the broad areas of structural, policy, and organizational changes as well as process change and patient preferences. His work also helped establish the systems approach to health care quality and its studies.

Quality as a business imperative evolved in the factory setting through specialization, mass production, and automation. In *Economic Control of Quality of Manufactured Product*, Shewhart points out that the goal should not be inspection and specifications but to minimize variation in processes and to focus on customer needs.[5] Influenced by his work with Shewhart, Deming recognized quality as a primary driver for business and communicated these methods to Japanese engineers and executives, which ultimately contributed to the tremendous successes in Japan in the 1950s and for years thereafter. Perhaps Deming's best known contribution to American industry is a set of management principles (Table 1-1) that are applicable in large or small organizations and in any business sector.[6] Deming's 14 Points constituted a second conceptual development that both followed and extended the Donabedian model. Quality management was redefined as not just a technical, clinical exercise but also as an issue of culture and values, psychological climate, and leadership—it provided another model for the improvement process.

In the 1980s and 1990s, the work of Crosby,[3] Deming,[6] and Juran[7] became well known in manufacturing across the United States. This work brought attention to systems design, process controls, and involvement of the entire workforce. Many executives who served on hospital and health system boards started using these concepts to push medical quality leaders to look beyond the boundaries of clinical quality assurance.

## TABLE 1-1 Deming's 14 Points

1. Create constancy of purpose toward improvement of product and service: the goal is to be competitive, to stay in business, and to provide jobs.

2. Adopt the new philosophy.

3. Cease dependence on inspection to achieve quality.

4. End the practice of awarding business on the basis of price tag. Instead, minimize total cost, move toward a single supplier for any one item, and build relationships based on loyalty and trust.

5. Improve constantly and forever the system of production and service, to improve quality and productivity, and thus decrease cost.

6. Institute training on the job.

7. Adopt and institute leadership: the goal is to help people and equipment do a better job.

8. Drive out fear, so that everyone may work effectively for the company.

9. Break down barriers between departments.

10. Eliminate slogans, exhortations, and targets for the workforce: asking for zero defects and new levels of productivity only creates adversarial relationships, as the bulk of the causes of low quality and low productivity belong to the system and thus lie beyond the power of the workforce.

11. a. Eliminate work standards (quotas) on the factory floor and substitute leadership;
    b. Eliminate management by objective; and
    c. Eliminate management by numbers and substitute leadership.

12. Remove barriers that rob the worker of his right to pride of workmanship. The responsibility of supervisors must be changed from sheer numbers to quality.

13. Institute a vigorous program of education and self-improvement.

14. Put everybody in the company to work to accomplish the transformation.

*Source:* Deming WE. *Out of the Crisis.* Cambridge, MA: MIT Press; 1986:23–24. Reprinted with permission from the MIT Press.

The boards were encouraged to consider all aspects of the health care organization as targets for improvement—from leadership style and behavior to the presence of information system support and collaboration between departments and disciplines. Clinical quality management was now seen as part of *total quality management* (TQM), which emphasizes that all members of the team possess a thorough understanding of the process and the knowledge of specific tools to assess and to improve processes (Table 1-2).[8] *Continuous quality improvement* (CQI), an important part of TQM, emphasizes the opportunity for improvement through continuous effort in every aspect of the organization's operations.

TABLE 1-2 Principles of Total Quality Management

The philosophy of TQM includes the following set of management principles:

1. CQI: a philosophy of continuously seeking improvement

2. Innovation: meeting customer needs in a whole new way

3. Quality into daily work life: integrating management principles into employee daily life

4. Strategic Quality Planning: the influence on long- and short-term planning

*Source:* Gustafson DH, Hundt AS. Findings of innovation research applied to quality management principles for health care. *Health Care Manage Rev.* 1995;20(2):16–33.

Concurrently during the 1980s and 1990s, various stakeholders (e.g., purchasers, regulators, patients, advocates) began to call for a more open examination of the quality of care. During these decades, health care professionals experienced a gradual erosion of autonomous quality control efforts. Accrediting bodies, such as the National Committee for Quality Assurance (NCQA) and the Joint Commission, as well as organizations like the National Quality Forum (NQF), became increasingly involved in the collection and assessment of quality data across the nation.

In 1998, Chassin and Galvin characterized the problems of overuse, underuse, and misuse in medicine and called attention to practice variation in medicine and to the suboptimal patient outcomes associated with this variation (Table 1-3).[9]

In 1999, Kohn, Corrigan, and Donaldson estimated that at least 75,000 people die from medical errors every year. Under their editorship, the IOM published *To Err Is Human: Building a Safer Health System* in 2000.[10] This report identified the systems that must be developed to decrease the number of medical errors in the United States. In a second report, *Crossing the Quality Chasm: A New Health System for the 21st Century*,[11] the IOM defined the state of the quality problem, offered recommendations for improvements, and outlined specific targets that would contribute to nationwide improvements (Table 1-4).

TABLE 1-3 Clinical Quality Problems in Health Services Provision

*Overuse:* The potential for harm from a health service exceeds the possible benefit.

*Underuse:* A health service that would have produced favorable outcomes was not provided.

*Misuse:* A preventable complication occurs with an appropriate service.

*Adapted from:* Chassin MR, Galvin RW. The urgent need to improve health care quality: Institute of Medicine National Roundtable on Health Care Quality. *JAMA.* 1998;280(11):1000–1005.

TABLE 1-4   **Recommendations from the First Two IOM Reports**

**To Err Is Human:**

- Establish a national focus to create leadership, research, tools, and protocols to enhance knowledge about safety.
- Learn from errors through immediate and strong mandatory reporting efforts.
- Create safety systems inside health care organizations through the implementation of safe practices at the delivery level.

**Crossing the Quality Chasm:**

Every health care system should be designed to provide care that is:

- *Safe*: avoid injury to patients from the care that is intended to help;
- *Effective*: provide services based on scientific knowledge to all who could benefit, and refrain from providing services to those not likely to benefit;
- *Patient-centered*: care that is responsive and respectful of individual patient preferences, needs, and values; ensure that patient values guide all clinical decisions;
- *Timely*: reduce wait time and harmful delays for both those who receive and those who give care;
- *Equitable*: provide care that does not vary in quality (i.e., care that is not influenced by personal characteristics such as gender, ethnicity, geographic location, and socioeconomic status).

*Sources:* Committee on Quality of Health Care in America, Institute of Medicine. Kohn LT, Corrigan JM, Donaldson MS, eds. *To Err Is Human: Building a Safer Health System*. Washington, DC: National Academies Press; 2000. And Committee on Quality of Health Care in America, Institute of Medicine. *Crossing the Quality Chasm: A New Health System for the 21st Century*. Washington, DC: National Academies Press; 2001.

## The Purpose and Philosophy of Quality Management

The purpose and philosophy of quality management has evolved from an orientation toward policing (i.e., finding "bad apples" among primarily excellent physicians, nurses, and clinical teams) to a focus on the use of quality management as a tool for continuous development of high performance.

Quality management can be thought of as having three aspects:

1. A means of *accountability* for the use of clinical and physical resources in the care of patients.

2. An effort to *continuously develop and improve* the services provided to patients by care teams throughout the organization and the community.

3. A mechanism to improve the *clinical outcomes of patients* as defined by the patient and the health care system.

Because the focus of quality management has broadened, quality management programs currently tend to target both *clinical* and *organizational structures* as well as *processes* that lead to improved outcomes.

Modern quality management leaders are systems thinkers, attending to both operating and strategic-level issues that concern quality. These quality management leaders put patients first, use data and information to examine and respond to problems, and rely on the participation of the entire workforce. They constantly seek changes that will co-produce improvement in a continuous cycle. Although outside regulators may check on the quality of care, the concerns of "outsiders" are dwarfed by the insiders' commitments to CQI of patient care systems and the outcomes they produce.

---

## CASE STUDY ● ● ●

### Using Continuous Quality Improvement to Decrease Mortality from Coronary Artery Bypass Graft Surgery

Using collaboration and CQI, the Northern New England Cardiovascular Disease Study Group, a voluntary regional consortium, achieved a 24% decline in mortality from coronary artery bypass graft (CABG) throughout the region.[12] This group included all cardiothoracic surgeons, interventional cardiologists, nurses, anesthesiologists, perfusionists, administrators, and scientists associated with the 6 medical centers in Maine, New Hampshire, and Vermont, and 1 Massachusetts-based medical center that supports CABG surgery and percutaneous coronary interventions. Training in CQI, benchmarking, and continued monitoring of outcomes allowed institutions to learn from one another. There were 293 fewer deaths ($n = 575$) than the 868 expected in the postintervention period (mid-1991 through early 1992). Major improvements in hospital outcomes have occurred in relation to improving coronary stenting technology. Variability in practice patterns across the different practices was a major stimulus to enhance quality of care across all sites.

---

## Implementing a Quality Improvement Project

Improvement projects often rise to the surface because of an adverse event or a patient or provider complaint, so there may not always be an opportunity to choose an improvement project. However, in instances when projects can be prioritized, reviewing potential improvement projects against the criteria depicted in Figures 1-1 and 1-2 may help identify the best QI projects to undertake first. In general, one would prefer projects that fit in quadrants I or II (Figure 1-1) and would avoid those with low impact. Clinical QI aims to enhance implementation of evidence-based medicine into clinical practice and to inform quality measurement with evidence-based process measures that are linked to outcomes. The Clinical Value Compass (Figure 1-2) developed by Nelson et al.[13] may be helpful to determine clinical QI projects that will have a maximal impact on outcomes.

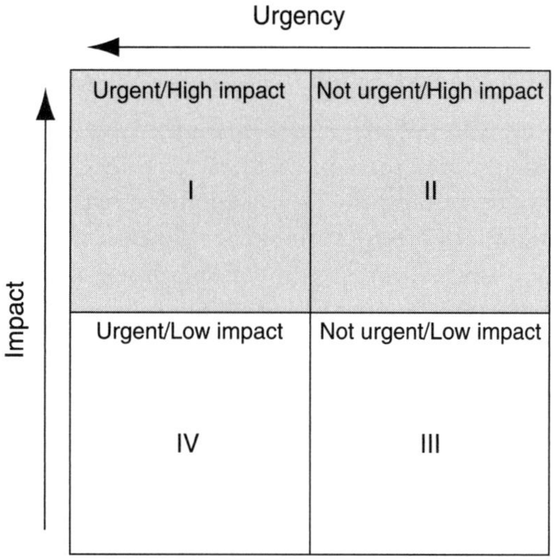

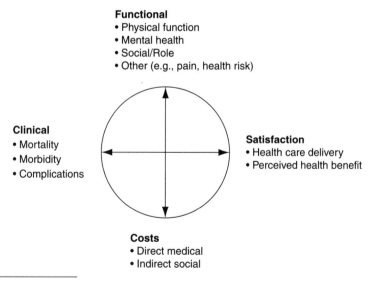

**Figure 1-1** Choosing a QI Project

*Source:* Bennet KE, Wichman R, Buntrock N, et al. *Choosing a QI Project.* Rochester, MN: Mayo Clinic, Division of Engineering, Project Prioritization Process; September 1999. Reprinted with permission of the Mayo Clinic, 2008.

Urgency

| Urgent/High impact | Not urgent/High impact |
| I | II |
| Urgent/Low impact | Not urgent/Low impact |
| IV | III |

Impact

**Functional**
• Physical function
• Mental health
• Social/Role
• Other (e.g., pain, health risk)

**Clinical**
• Mortality
• Morbidity
• Complications

**Satisfaction**
• Health care delivery
• Perceived health benefit

**Costs**
• Direct medical
• Indirect social

**Figure 1-2** Clinical Value Compass

*Source:* Nelson EC, Mohr JJ, Batalden PB, Plume SK. Improving health care, part 1: The clinical value compass. *Jt Comm J Qual Improv.* 1996;22(4):243–258. © Joint Commission Resources. Reprinted with permission.

## Tools for Quality Improvement

### Process Mapping

Regardless of the improvement methodology used, once a QI project is chosen, a systematic process, perhaps best described by the Seven-Step Model,[14] detailed in Figure 1-3, is key to guiding the project implementation. Step 3, which includes process mapping, is a key, yet often overlooked, step that is crucial to understanding an existing clinical or system process. Process mapping involves studying the entire process through various techniques including photography or videotaping, observation ("fly on the wall"),

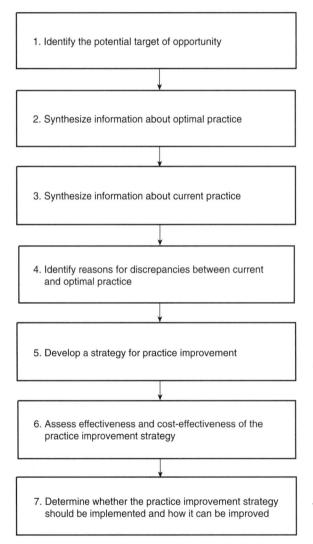

**Figure 1-3** Seven-Step Model for Process Improvement

*Source:* Matchar DB, Samsa GP. The role of evidence reports in evidence-based medicine: A mechanism for linking scientific evidence and practice improvement. *Jt Comm J Qual Improv.* 1999;25(10): 522–528. © Joint Commission Resources. Reprinted with permission.

interviewing, field notes, and role play as necessary. The process map can then be depicted by using flow charts.

## Flow Charts

These charts allow for identification of the alignment of processes that must be followed in the QI project. They identify the beginning and the end of the process and how one part of the process is dependent on another. Table 1-5 is a matrix for the use of flow charts and Figure 1-4 is an example of a flow chart.

## Cause-and-Effect (Fishbone) Diagram

Another common tool used in QI projects is the cause-and-effect diagram, also referred to as a fishbone or Ishikawa diagram, which can be used to enhance the QI team's ability to map the full range of possible root contributors to the desired outcome. A *fishbone diagram* is a graphical representation of relationships among the fundamental variables on which the group will focus when initiating improvement action (Figure 1-5). The diagram is used to expand the group's purview and to begin to generate consensus on targets for action. It is commonly used to analyze sentinel events and is described in more detail in Chapter 3.

---

**TABLE 1-5    Matrix for Use of Flow Charts**

**What does this method do?**
Allows a team to identify the actual flow or sequence of events in a process that any product or service follows.

**Why use this method?**
Shows unexpected complexity, problem areas, redundancy, and unnecessary loops, and reveals areas where simplification and standardization may be possible.

Compares and contrasts the actual versus the ideal flow of a process to identify improvement opportunities.

Allows a team to come to an agreement on the steps of the process and to examine which activities may impact the process performance.

Identifies locations where additional data can be collected and researched.

Serves as a training aid for understanding and completing the process.

**How do you effectively use this method?**
Identify the boundaries of the process. Clearly define where the process under discussion begins and ends.

Team members should agree on the level of detail they must show on the flow chart to clearly understand the process and identify problem areas.

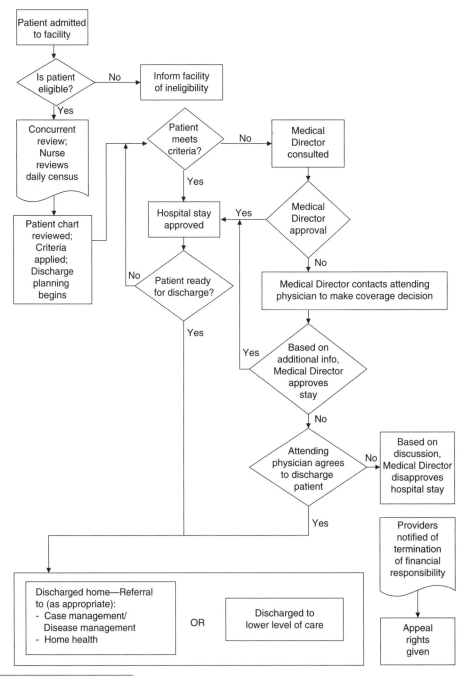

**Figure 1-4** Example of a Flow Chart for Admission

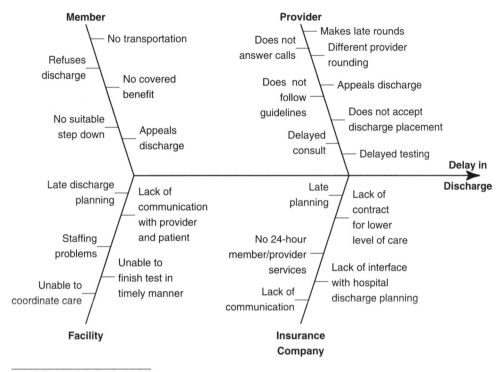

**Figure 1-5**   Example of a Fish Bone Diagram Illustrating Late Discharge from a Hospital

## Brainstorming and Affinity Diagrams

The technique of storyboarding grew out of the film and cartoon industry; Disney Studios perfected it to an art form. In planning and organizational work, storyboarding is more properly called an *affinity diagram*. The process begins with brainstorming, during which every participant writes ideas about addressing a given issue on separate cards and mounts those cards on a large corkboard or similar display (the storyboard). During the ensuing discussion, the ideas are grouped according to subject matter—hence the term affinity diagram. Further discussion enables the participants to rearrange the groups into clusters, to identify subject headings, and to identify them as causes, symptoms, impacts, or side effects of the original issue. The affinity diagram that results from the brainstorming session is typically used at the beginning of a QI project or process. If affinity diagramming occurs later in the process, when individuals or group members are identifying actions for addressing immediate problems, the diagram will most likely contain alternatives that the group members have identified as actions to take. Table 1-6 describes brainstorming, and Table 1-7 explains how affinity diagrams are used.

TABLE 1-6   Creating Great Ideas by Brainstorming

**What does this method do?**

Provides a way of creatively and efficiently generating a high volume of ideas on any topic by creating a process that is free of criticism and judgment.

**Why use this method?**

Encourages open thinking and teamwork.

Involves all team members.

Allows team members to build on each other's creativity while maintaining a unified goal.

**How do you effectively use this method?**

For clarity, state the question to be discussed and write it down.

Allow everyone to offer ideas without criticism!

Write each idea down, to be visible to all team members.

Review the list of ideas for clarity and to discard duplicates.

Participants may build on ideas of others.

## Pareto Chart

Once themes and clusters of potential causes of a lack of quality in an area of care have been noted, the factors contributing most to the problem must be identified. Without inspecting the data, managers may assume that all causes contribute equally to poor quality or that one or more causes are the leading ones. *Pareto diagrams*, often expressed as bar graphs, help show the relative contribution of the various causes of the problem.

TABLE 1-7   Gathering and Grouping Ideas in an Affinity Diagram

**What does this method do?**

Allows a team to organize and summarize ideas after a brainstorming session to better understand the essence of a problem and to possibly reach breakthrough solutions.

**Why use this method?**

Encourages creativity by all team members at all phases of the process.

Encourages creative connectivity of ideas and issues.

Allows breakthrough solutions to emerge naturally (even on long-standing issues).

Encourages participant ownership of results.

**How do you effectively use this method?**

Phrase the issue under discussion in a clear and complete sentence.

Brainstorm at least 20 ideas and issues and record each on sticky notes.

Sort ideas into related groups of 5 to 10 ideas.

Create summary or header cards using the consensus for each group.

TABLE 1-8   Using a Pareto Chart

**What does this method do?**
Expends efforts on problems that offer the best possible improvement by showing their relative
frequency or size in a descending bar graph.

**Why use this method?**
Helps a team to focus on causes that will have the greatest impact if solved.
Based on the Pareto principle: 20% of the sources cause 80% of any problem.
Helps prevent "shifting the problem"; the "solution" removes some causes but worsens others.

**How do you effectively use this method?**
Decide which problem you want to know more about.
Categorize the causes or problems that will be monitored, compared, and ranked by brain-
storming or with existing data.
Choose the most meaningful unit of measurement, such as frequency or cost.
Choose the time period for the study.
Collect the key data on each problem category either by "real time" or by reviewing
historical data.
Compare the relative frequency or cost of each problem category.
List problem categories on the horizontal line and frequencies on the vertical line.
Interpret the results: Tallest bars indicate the largest contributors to the overall problem.

Table 1-8 describes the use of Pareto charts, and Figure 1-6 presents a Pareto chart that
was developed to help a provider group examine its late discharges from a hospital.

## Histogram

The *histogram* can help elucidate the reasons for a variation by depicting the frequency
of each value of the quantitative variable. For example, the first step in understanding
the reasons for variation in hospital discharge times is to choose a sample time span,
perhaps a 2-week period, and to count the number of patients who were discharged each
hour during that period. The values can then be graphed on a histogram (Table 1-9 and
Figure 1-7).

## Bar Chart

A *bar chart* is similar to a histogram, except that the variable of interest is not a quantitative measure, such as discharge time, but rather a categorical variable, such as a department within the hospital. Bar charts are commonly used to illustrate comparisons, such
as the number of patients discharged before or after 11:00 a.m. for each of several hospital
services, and may help identify departments that require further attention. As with
histograms, bar charts are especially useful for diagnosis and evaluation. A bar chart that

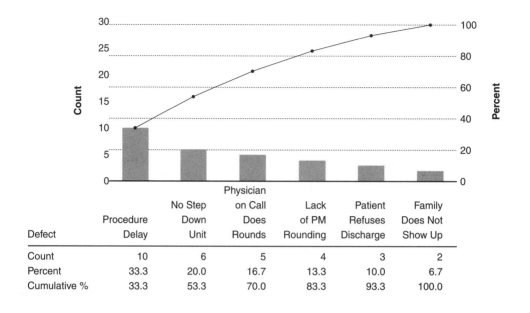

| Defect | Procedure Delay | No Step Down Unit | Physician on Call Does Rounds | Lack of PM Rounding | Patient Refuses Discharge | Family Does Not Show Up |
|---|---|---|---|---|---|---|
| Count | 10 | 6 | 5 | 4 | 3 | 2 |
| Percent | 33.3 | 20.0 | 16.7 | 13.3 | 10.0 | 6.7 |
| Cumulative % | 33.3 | 53.3 | 70.0 | 83.3 | 93.3 | 100.0 |

**Figure 1-6** Example of a Pareto Chart to Examine Reasons for Delayed Discharge from a Hospital

---

**TABLE 1-9 Using a Histogram to Achieve Process Centering, Spread, and Shape**

**What does this method do?**

Aids in making decisions about a process or product that could be improved after examining the variation.

**Why use this method?**

Displays measurement data in bar graph format, distributed in categories.

Displays large amounts of data that are not easily interpreted in tabular form.

Shows the relative frequency of occurrence of the various data values.

Depicts the centering, variation, and shape of the data for easy interpretation.

Helps to indicate if the process has changed.

Displays the variation in the process quite easily.

**How do you effectively use this method?**

Gather and tabulate data on a process, product, or procedure (e.g., time, weight, size, frequency of occurrences, test scores, GPAs, pass/fail rates, number of days to complete a cycle).

Calculate the rate of the data by subtracting the smallest number in the data set from the largest. Call this value R.

*(continues)*

**TABLE 1-9**  *continued*

Decide about how many bars (or classes) to display in the eventual histogram. Call this number K. This number should never be less than four and seldom exceeds 12. With 100 numbers, K = 7 generally works well. With 1000 pieces of data, K = 11 works well.

Determine the fixed width of each class by dividing the range, R, by the number of classes, K. This value should be rounded to a "nice" number, generally a number ending in a zero. For example, 11.3 would not a "nice" number, but 10 would. Call this number I, for interval width. The use of "nice" numbers avoids strange scales on the x-axis of the histogram.

Create a table of upper and lower class limits. Add the interval width to the first "nice" number less the lowest value in the data set to determine the upper limit of the first class.

The first "nice" number becomes the lowest lower limit of the first class. The upper limit of the first becomes the lower limit of the second class. Adding the interval width (I) to the lower limit of the second class determines the upper limit for the second class. Repeat this process until the largest upper limit exceeds the largest data piece. You should have approximate classes or categories in total.

Plot the frequency data on the histogram framework by drawing vertical bars for each class. The height of each bar represents the number.

Note the frequency of values between the lower and upper limits of that particular class.

Interpret the histogram for skew and clustering problems.

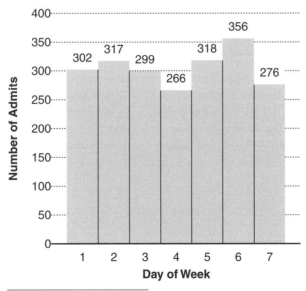

**Figure 1-7**  Example of a Histogram

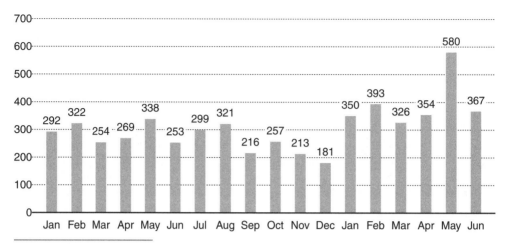

**Figure 1-8**    Example of a Bar Chart of Lab Tests by Month

displays the number of laboratory tests performed by a physician group by month is shown in Figure 1-8.

## Scatter Diagram

The *scatter diagram* in Figure 1-9 shows the relationship between length of stay (LOS) and time of discharge and examines whether there is a pattern to this relationship; if so, the QI team could then investigate whether the pattern was controllable. Table 1-10 explains the method and use of a scatter diagram.

## Statistical Control Chart

Processes typically have two kinds of variation; normal variation that occurs under normal conditions and abnormal variation that occurs under unusual circumstances and often can be traced to a cause. A *statistical control chart* represents continuous application of a particular statistical decision rule to distinguish between normal and abnormal variations. Statistical control charts have been widely used to control quality in the management process. The use of a statistical control chart is further explained in Chapter 2.

# Methods for Quality Improvement

While there are several methods for quality improvement, we will focus on the three that are most commonly used in health care. Each has common elements and varies slightly for different settings, all eventually leading to testing and change. More recently, principles from different methodologies are being used for the same project, making their differences less relevant (e.g., use of Sigma-Lean methodology).[15]

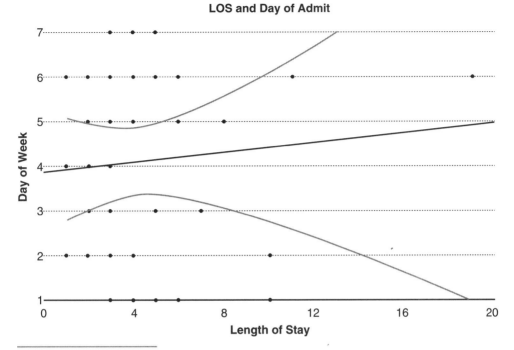

**Figure 1-9** Example of a Scatter Diagram Showing Correlation Between Length of Stay and Day of Admission

---

**TABLE 1-10   Using a Scatter Diagram to Measure Relationships Between Variables**

**What does this method do?**

Analyzes and identifies the possible relationship between the changes observed in two different measurements.

**Why use this method?**

Provides the data to confirm a hypothesis.

Depicts both visual and statistical means to test the strength of a potential relationship.

Provides a good follow-up to a cause-and-effect diagram to determine if more than a consensus connection exists between causes and the effect.

**How do you effectively use this method?**

Collect the data (50–100 paired samples of related data) and construct a data sheet.

Draw the x-axis and the y-axis, and plot points corresponding to these measures for each observation.

Interpret the data to determine if any pattern or trend emerges, noting positive or negative correlation.

## Plan, Do, Study, Act (PDSA) Methodology

This process is also referred to as the *Shewhart cycle*, or *PDSA* (Plan, Do, Study, Act) *methodology*. It involves a trial-and-learning methodology whereby a hypothesis or suggested solution for improvement is made and tested on a small scale before any changes are made to the whole system.[16] A logical sequence of four repetitive steps (Figure 1-10) are carried out over a course of small cycles, which eventually leads to exponential improvements (Figure 1-11).

During the *Plan* stage of the Shewhart cycle, the areas in need of QI are identified. These can be high-cost, high-volume, high-risk areas, or areas in which outcome results are not as good as the organization would like. This part of the cycle involves developing indicators and monitors, thresholds and benchmarks, and the methodology for the study intervention. The *Do* part of the cycle entails implementation and documenting problems and unexpected observations. The *Study* portion of the cycle involves collecting data from the *Do* part of the cycle and then producing information from those data. The final stage of the cycle, *Act*, involves determining whether the intervention produced improved outcomes as reflected in the information. If the intervention did produce

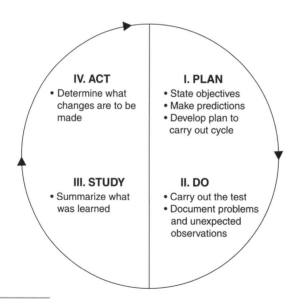

**Figure 1-10**   The PDSA Cycle

*Sources:* Berwick DM. Developing and testing changes in delivery of care. *Ann Int Med.* 1998;128(8): 651–656. And Langley GJ, Nolan KM, et al. *The Improvement Guide* (Figure 1-1). Hackensack, NJ: Jossey-Bass; 1996. Reprinted with permission from Wiley/Jossey-Bass.

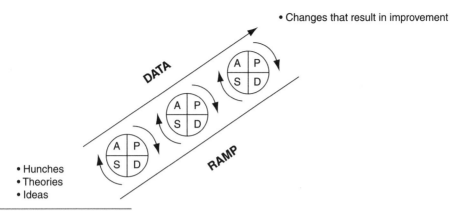

**Figure 1-11** Ramp of Improvement: A Sequence of Multiple PDSA Cycles

*Source:* Langley GJ, Nolan KM, et al. *The Improvement Guide* (Figure 1-3). Hackensack, NJ: Jossey-Bass; 1996. Reprinted with permission from Wiley/Jossey-Bass.

improved outcomes, it may be continued to determine whether improvement can be maintained; if it did not produce improved outcomes, the cycle begins anew, and a new intervention is tried. The tools of data analysis and presentation described previously are used at one or more points in this problem-solving process.

*Nolan's Three-Question Model* is often used at the start of a project to determine the aim for the project, to establish measures, and to select changes.[17] The aim of the project should be time specific and measurable; the measures chosen are quantifiable and determine if a specific change actually leads to an improvement. The changes that are most likely to result in improvement are chosen and tested through the PDSA cycles (Figure 1-12).

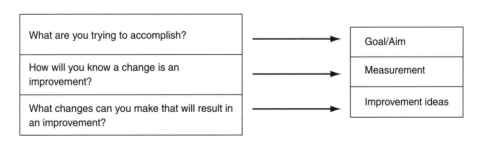

**Figure 1-12** Nolan's Three-Question Model

*Adapted from:* Langley GJ, Nolan KM, et al. *The Improvement Guide* (Figure 1-13). Hackensack, NJ: Jossey-Bass; 1996. Reprinted with permission from Wiley/Jossey-Bass.

## Six Sigma

Sigma is the 18th letter of the Greek alphabet and the symbol for standard deviation. It is now utilized in service and health care organizations. The aim of *Six Sigma* is to reach a level of quality that resides in the 6 standard deviations of average performance, resulting in an error rate of 0.0003% or about 3.4 defects per million opportunities; at this stage the process is virtually error free (99.9996%).[18]

Six Sigma uses data to identify quality problems, or potential quality problems, and areas for improvement. The Six Sigma approach concentrates on customer-driven measures and acceptable quality and relies on data-driven process improvement. Six Sigma is achieved through a series of steps (akin to the PDSA cycle) identified as define, measure, analyze, improve, and control (DMAIC). Six Sigma is generally instituted by practitioners, known as Six Sigma Black Belts, who have been trained in the use of the proper analytic tools to address quality problems. A certified Black Belt understands and can effectively employ DMAIC, demonstrates team leadership, understands team dynamics, and is able to assign team member roles and responsibilities appropriately.

The first step of the DMAIC model entails the *Definition* of the problem, the project parameters, and the establishment of an improvement objective. In the second step, *Measure*, the measurement of each of the process steps is conducted and data collected. In the third step, an *Analysis* of the collected data is performed to test a hypothesis about key process factors. In the fourth step, the process is *Improved* by conducting a pilot test. In the final step of the cycle, the process is *Controlled* by implementing the process improvement and continuously working to monitor and sustain the process.

For Six Sigma efforts to be successful, senior management must support them. These efforts cut across operational lines, use the most talented people in the organization, and move them into new areas. The Six Sigma concept is expected to become more popular in health care organizations over the next several years. It is especially useful for processes that are repeated in large numbers (e.g., laboratory tests, radiological procedures).

---

## CASE STUDY ● ● ●

### *Use of Six Sigma to Reduce Process Variations and Costs in Radiology*

The Commonwealth Health Corporation (CHC) in Bowling Green, Kentucky, is a not-for-profit integrated delivery network that includes 3 medical centers and 1 extended care facility with over 2000 employees. Six Sigma was implemented within the Radiology Department in early 1998. Department members were trained in the Six Sigma approach, and participants achieved Green Belt status. At the completion of projects progressed Green Belts to Black Belts and then to Master Black Belt status. As a result, the Radiology project reduced wait times for patients, generated faster turnaround times for radiology reports, and increased productivity. CHC's team managed to increase throughput by 25% while using fewer resources and decreasing costs per radiology procedure by 21.5%. In total, radiology cost/procedure decreased from $68.13 to $49.55 for the over 100,000 procedures a year, resulting in a $1.65 million cumulative savings. In addition, errors in magnet resonance imaging (MRIs) decreased by 90% resulting in a cost savings of $800,000 within the 18-month period.[19]

## Lean

*Lean methodology* is used to accelerate the velocity and reduce the cost of any process by removing any type of activity that absorbs resources and yet creates no value (also known as *muda*).[20] Perhaps the most noted and benchmarked "lean" organization is Toyota Manufacturing of Japan. Several health care systems have used Toyota's process (also called the Toyota Production System or TPS) to improve health care quality in their organization.[21]

One of the common terms used in Lean is *Kaizen*, a Japanese word meaning gradual and orderly continuous improvement. Kaizen is essentially a rapid, relatively low-cost, simple, team-based approach to improvement. A *Kaizen Blitz* or a *Kaizen Event* is an intense process for introducing rapid change into a work unit or organization using the ideas, the motivation, and the energy of the people who do the work. The general principles and approaches behind Kaizen that are potentially very useful to health care quality improvement are described in Table 1-11.

Lean thinking improves process outcomes by removing non-value-added processes including the waste of overproduction and underproduction (e.g., smoothing day-to-day variations in radiological procedures), waste of inventory (e.g., excess patient IV pumps in storage), waste of rework–rejects (e.g., poorly done lab tests), waste of motion (e.g., repeating several steps to obtain clinical data from a medical record), waste of waiting (e.g., patients waiting for appointments), waste of processing (e.g., decreasing steps in the

---

TABLE 1-11    **Some Tenets of Kaizen**

1. Discard conventional fixed ideas.

2. Think of how to solve a problem, not why it cannot be done.

3. Do not make excuses to start a project. Start by questioning current practices.

4. Do not seek perfection; implement solutions even if it will only achieve 50% of target.

5. Correct a mistake right away.

6. Use wisdom for problem solving, not money.

7. Ask "why?" five times and seek root causes.

8. Seek the wisdom of 10 people rather than the knowledge of one.

9. Use the wisdom of frontline employees.

*Adapted from:* Womack J, Jones D. *Lean Thinking: Banish Waste and Create Wealth in Your Company.* New York: Simon & Schuster (Free Press); 2003.

emergency department admission process), and waste of transporting (e.g., unnecessary transfer of patients between patient care units). In addition, lean processes line up value-creating steps in the best possible sequence in order to deliver services or products just as the customer needs them and in just the manner the customer requested. One of the most commonly used tools is called *Value Stream Mapping* whereby the process is depicted in a physical graph in order to identify wasted effort or steps that do not add value for the customer.

The three QI methods discussed are summarized and compared in Table 1-12.

## Commonly Used Quality Improvement Strategies

Most published literature suggests the use of multipronged approaches for successful QI as opposed to single interventions. Descriptions of commonly used QI strategies follow.

### Academic Detailing

*Academic detailing*, also called *educational outreach*, employs trained providers (e.g., pharmacists, physicians) to conduct face-to-face visits to encourage adoption of a desired

| TABLE 1-12 | Comparison of Improvement Methodologies | | |
|---|---|---|---|
| | **PDSA** | **Six Sigma** | **Lean** |
| Process Steps | Plan; Do; Study; Act. | Design; Measure; Analyze; Improve; Control. | Eliminate non-value–laden steps; eliminate defects; reduce cycle time. |
| Improvement Focus | Rapid cycles of improvement toward identifying optimal process improvement. | Elimination of defects; customer-centric. | Enhanced efficiency; elimination of non-value activities, variance reduction and reduced cycle time. Product "flows" when the customer wants and needs it. |
| Ideal Use | A target project is chosen for improvement; time and resources are limited. | A targeted project is chosen for improvement and resources are available. The project consists of an activity that is repeated with high frequency. | Process efficiency is the focus. Process can be clearly defined and is laden with non-value activities. |
| Supports–Tools for success | Environment for testing, prototyping, and piloting of ideas. | Statistical process control charts, analytical tools, Six Sigma experts (i.e., black belts, green belts). | Value stream mapping, value analysis, Kaizen events. |

behavior pattern. Although academic detailing was originally conceived and proven effective as a one-on-one educational intervention, several studies have incorporated academic detailing principles in small group sessions. Academic detailing has been shown to be effective at enhancing provider knowledge and changing prescribing behaviors, although it has generally been proven ineffective at enhancing patient outcomes in a sustained fashion.[22]

## Opinion Leaders

*Opinion leaders* are members of the local system who are usually able to influence others either on a broad range of issues or in a single area of acknowledged expertise. They do not always have leadership titles, but they generally have higher status among their peers and higher visibility. Peer feedback from local opinion leaders has been shown to have a modest effect on enhancing quality of care and has been used as part of multifaceted QI strategies in several institutions.[23]

## Audit and Feedback

This strategy entails the provision of a summary of the clinical performance of an individual provider, practice, or clinic to the respective entity. It is often done in conjunction with reports that contain anonymous performance rates of comparable clinics or providers. Based on the timeliness and type of feedback, this strategy has shown small to modest benefits in the improvement of targeted processes or outcomes, especially when combined with achievable benchmark feedback. In a study of diabetes patients by Kiefe et al.,[23] physicians were randomly assigned to receive either a chart review and physician-specific feedback or an identical intervention plus achievable benchmark feedback. Odds ratios for patients of the achievable benchmark physicians versus comparison physicians were higher for influenza vaccination, foot examination, lipid control, and long-term glucose control measurement.

## Reminder Systems

These interventions prompt providers to remember information relevant to a particular encounter, patient, or service. They are often effective when integrated into the work flow and are available at the point of care delivery. An example is the system of flagging charts of patients whose influenza vaccinations are due, which prompts the provider to remember and enhances recommendation of influenza vaccination at the time of the visit.

## Patient Education

Individual or group sessions to enhance patient self-management of disease were shown to have modest to large effects based on patient characteristics and conditions. These effects have been well studied, especially in the management of diabetes mellitus and chronic heart failure.

## Case Management

*Case management* and disease management are described in detail in Chapter 7. They are well-studied QI strategies used to manage special populations who have specific diagnoses or who require high-cost or intensive services. These services are often centralized and involve coordination of health care interventions and communications for members. This strategy has demonstrated a positive effect on enhancing quality of care for patients with chronic diseases.

## Reengineering

*Reengineering* and process redesign consist of improving an existing process or system in such a way that allows expanded opportunities to be met or existing problems to be solved. This broadens the reach by allowing additional uses, generating lower costs, or delivering improvements in usability. Because of the nature of the process, this strategy has often yielded novel product or service innovations that go beyond the realm of improvement and result in the redesign of existing structures and/or processes. Examples are the use of telemedicine to enhance access to care in remote locations or convenient care clinics to enhance access and efficiency and to create new business models for health care service.

## Incentives

This strategy is described in detail in Chapter 6. Financial incentives for achieving a certain percentage increase or target level of compliance with targeted processes of care have shown evidence of achieving target goals. This concept has led to the current strategy of pay-for-performance. There is less evidence that negative incentives such as withholding of salary or year-end bonuses for not achieving target performance are an effective means of enhancing quality of care.

# Quality Improvement Research

There is often confusion about whether a project is purely QI or research. In general, QI is used when changes need to be made to a local system for clinical management. In this case, the effects of rapid changes are studied using small samples and less rigorous documentation; this provides for rapid feedback to the system. A project is considered QI research if (1) there is deviation from established good practices, (2) the subjects are individual patients rather than systems or providers, (3) randomization or blinding is conducted, (4) the majority of the patients are not expected to benefit directly from the knowledge gained, and/or (5) participants are subject to interventions that are not required in routine care.

There is limited understanding of the factors that truly make a QI project successful because systems changes often have multiple confounding factors, thus creating an urgent need for rigorous research in this area. It is especially important to know the costs of the intervention, any possible unintended "side effects" of the intervention, if the intervention contributed to improved patient outcomes in addition to improving the process, and if the overall effect of individual QI efforts actually enhances the quality of the entire system. As Perneger suggests, it is important to keep in mind that although quality improvement is the aim, not all change may be an improvement.[24]

Study designs that may be useful in QI research include randomized controlled trials, controlled studies, pre- and postintervention studies, as well as time series. Rigorous research designs become especially important when results are to be generalized and/or communicated externally, and the impact of the change is potentially large.

## Challenges to Successful Quality Improvement

Many organizations have encountered difficulties when implementing quality management. Barriers may be found in the organization's technology, structure, psychological climate, leadership, culture, and involvement in legal issues. A summary of each of these areas is described below.

### Technology

Many organizations' quality managers have had to learn new quality management techniques while simultaneously building the information infrastructure needed to do the work. In many organizations, the technology of quality management is relatively new and has only been lightly used and tested by the staff. Many technological innovations still await widespread diffusion due to a lack of necessary resources and change management necessary for implementation.

### Structure

Some leaders have taken aggressive steps to put quality councils in place, to recognize QI gains in public ways, and to inject quality into performance requirements; however, these efforts are by no means widespread. How to structure the quality effort and how much visibility to give the quality initiative in the organizational structure are two barriers that often result in inaction.

### Psychological Climate

The climate of the organization sometimes presents a barrier to two fundamental aspects of quality philosophy: openness to data sharing and teamwork. Quality management requires that the staff collect and analyze data and share the findings transparently in open meetings, yet the climate of some organizations is too closed for this type of exposure. In other organizations, teamwork is only an occasional proposition. Because QI depends on examining relationships and interdependencies across departmental boundaries and hierarchical levels, a lack of familiarity with this "boundary-less" movement may be a barrier.

## Leadership

Just as leadership can support quality management, it can also obstruct it. Unless quality management has a clear and continuous commitment from the organization's leader, the quality effort is doomed. Frequently, the leader fails to adequately communicate the importance of the quality effort and its ongoing progress. The leader must constantly demonstrate visible support for the quality effort. Clinical and administrative staffs are keenly sensitive to any real or perceived wavering of support.

## Culture

In Deming's view,[6] successful quality management requires building a supportive organizational culture. Conversely, an organizational culture that has the following characteristics conflicts with the basic philosophy of quality management: decisions are made from the top down; the workforce is not empowered; communication tends to be closed (i.e., data are not openly shared); patients' interests are subservient to medical center objectives; errors bring blame-seeking and dismissal; and teamwork is thought to be unnecessary. Initiating quality efforts in a hostile environment is a doomed experiment. Unfortunately, many academic medical centers and large community institutions lack a history of a supportive culture for QI.

## Legal Issues

An easy way to disable a quality program is to saddle it with legal implications. In such a climate, patients will not sign release forms, and the organization cannot legally ask for or disseminate information related to quality or safety. Because provider contracts do not specify that data can be requested, an organization's managers must be creative and innovative in moving these legal issues aside without harming the organization, its employees, and the patients who receive care.

# Future Trends

The IOM reports heightened public and industry awareness of medical errors and quality issues in the health care system. Accrediting bodies and regulations have prompted health care institutions to enhance their QI and quality measurement initiatives to address these issues, resulting in a renewed interest in QI across the nation. Similarly, accrediting bodies of health professions education are increasingly interested in establishing competencies for upcoming graduates in the areas of QI and safety. This has resulted in a proliferation of curricula including early involvement of trainees in QI efforts to enhance patient care.

The past decade has seen surging interest in public reporting of sentinel events, as well as performance and outcome data of health care institutions. The Centers for Medicare and Medicaid Services (CMS) has already announced pay-for-performance initiatives, as well as plans to withhold payment for several adverse events not found to be present on admission.

Health care providers armed with knowledge of QI will be key to the success of such initiatives and shaping policy in this area, especially if they are supported by regulations that impose consequences to achieve compliance and accountability.

## References

1. Codman EA. The product of a hospital. *Surg Gynecol Obstet.* 1914;18:491–496.
2. Your guide to choosing quality health care: a quick look at quality. http://www.ahrq.gov/consumer/qnt/qntqlook.htm. Accessed July 16, 2006.
3. Crosby PB. *Quality Is Free: The Art of Making Quality Certain.* New York: McGraw-Hill; 1979.
4. Donabedian A. *The Methods and Findings of Quality Assessment and Monitoring.* Vols I, II, III. Ann Arbor, MI: Health Administration Press; 1985.
5. Shewhart W. *Economic Control of Quality of Manufactured Product.* New York: D. Van Nostrand Co.; 1931.
6. Deming WE. *Out of the Crisis.* Cambridge, MA: MIT Press; 1986:23–24.
7. Juran JM. *Juran on Leadership for Quality.* New York: Free Press; 1989.
8. Gustafson DH, Hundt AS. Findings of innovation research applied to quality management principles for health care. *Health Care Management Rev.* 1995;20(2):16–33.
9. Chassin MR, Galvin RW. The urgent need to improve health care quality. Institute of Medicine National Roundtable on Health Care Quality. *JAMA.* 1998;280(11):1000–1005.
10. Committee on Quality of Health Care in America, Institute of Medicine. Kohn LT, Corrigan JM, Donaldson MS, eds. *To Err Is Human: Building a Safer Health System.* Washington, DC: National Academies Press; 2000.
11. Committee on Quality of Health Care in America, Institute of Medicine. *Crossing the Quality Chasm: A New Health System for the 21st Century.* Washington, DC: National Academies Press; 2001.
12. Malenka DJ, O'Connor GT. A regional collaborative effort for CQI in cardiovascular disease: Northern New England Cardiovascular Study Group. *Jt Comm J Qual Improv.* 1995;21(11):627–633.
13. Nelson EC, Mohr JJ, Batalden PB, Plume SK. Improving health care, part 1: The clinical value compass. *Jt Comm J Qual Improv.* 1996;22(4):243–258.
14. Matchar DB, Samsa GP. The role of evidence reports in evidence-based medicine. *Jt Comm J Qual Improv.* 1999;25(10):522–528.
15. Varkey P, Reller MK, Resar R. The basics of quality improvement in healthcare. *Mayo Clin Proc.* 2007;82(6):735–739.
16. Berwick DM. Developing and testing changes in delivery of care. *Ann Intern Med.* 1998;128(8):651–656.
17. Langley GJ, Nolan KM, Nolan TW, et al. *The Improvement Guide.* San Francisco, CA: Jossey-Bass; 1996.
18. Goldstein M. Six Sigma program success factors. *Six Sigma Forum Magazine.* 2001 Nov: 36–45.
19. Cherry J, Seshadri S. Using statistics to reduce process variability and costs in radiology. *Radiology Mgmt.* 2000;8(1):42–45.
20. Womack J, Jones D. *Lean Thinking: Banish Waste and Create Wealth in Your Corporation.* New York: Simon and Schuster; 1996.

21. Young D. Pittsburgh hospitals band together to reduce medication errors. *Am J Health Syst Pharm.* 2002;59(11):1014, 1016, 1026.

22. Goldberg HI, Wagner EH, Fihn SD, et al. A randomized controlled trial of CQI teams and academic detailing: Can they alter compliance with guidelines? *Jt Comm J Qual Improv.* 1998;24(3):130–142.

23. Kiefe CI, Allison JJ, Williams OD, et al. Improving quality improvement using achievable benchmarks for physician feedback. *JAMA.* 2001;285:2871–2879.

24. Perneger TV. Why we need ethical oversight of quality improvement projects. *Int J Qual Health Care.* 2004;16(5):343–344.

## Additional Resources–Further Reading

Agency for Healthcare Research and Quality: http://www.ahrq.gov
Joint Commission: http://www.jointcommission.org
National Committee for Quality Assurance: http://www.ncqa.org
National Quality Forum: http://www.qualityforum.org
Quality and Safety in Healthcare: http://www.qhc.bmjjournals.com
Medicare (Centers for Medicare and Medicaid Services): http://www.medicare.gov
National Association for Healthcare Quality: http://www.nahq.org
American Health Quality Association: http://www.ahqa.org
Institute for Healthcare Improvement: http://www.ihi.org
Foundation for Health Care Quality: http://www.qualityhealth.org
FACCT (Foundation for Accountability): http://www.facct.org
Health Resources and Services Administration: http://www.ask.hrsa.gov/quality.cfm
Institute of Medicine Quality Initiative: http://www.iom.edu/?id=19174
American College of Medical Quality: http://www.acmq.org
Utilization Review Accreditation Commission (URAC): http://www.urac.org
Quality Interagency Coordination Task Force (QuIC): http://www.quic.gov
RAND Health: http://www.rand.org/health
Kaiser Family Foundation: http://www.kaisernetwork.org

# Chapter 2

# Quality Measurement

*Linda Harrington, PhD, RN, CNS, CPHQ, and*

*Harry Pigman, MD, MSHP*

## Executive Summary

Measurement is fundamental to any attempt to assess or to improve the quality and safety of health care. The history of measurement of health care quality parallels the history of epidemiology and statistics in the late 19th and early 20th centuries and is intertwined with the evolution of health services research in the late 20th century. Fortunately, only basic knowledge of these subjects is required by the typical clinician or administrator striving to improve health care. This chapter will focus on those concepts necessary for the practical application of measurement in QI.

### *Learning Objectives*

Upon completion of this chapter, readers should be able to:

- discuss the historical evolution of the science of quality measurement;
- compare and contrast the characteristics of structure, process, and outcome measurements;
- construct appropriate measurements for QI projects;
- discuss the necessary characteristics of quality measures, including reliability and validity;
- evaluate the success of QI projects; and
- identify upcoming trends in the science of quality measurement.

## History

The science of quality measurement is commonly recognized to have originated in the work of Florence Nightingale and her reports to the British parliament on mortality rates in British field hospitals during the Crimean War. Her early efforts to quantify health care were coupled with the birth of modern concepts of infection control, giving credence to the idea that measurement is needed for improvement.[1]

Several decades later, Ernest Codman[2,3] linked the interest in mortality to invasive procedures. His exploration of postsurgical mortality can be considered the start of investigations into hospital outcomes. Codman also is credited with the notions that hospitals should have organized medical staffs and records of patient care—essentially the birth of structural measures.

The next major development in the measurement of quality occurred outside of health care in the interval between the World Wars. Walter Shewhart[4] developed a branch of new statistics called statistical process control while working on the manufacture of telephones. Perhaps his most important contribution was a change in the focus of measurement from the quality of products themselves to the steps required to produce those products. His other major contribution was a method to identify shifts in the manufacturing process that were statistically meaningful, a method that was simple enough to be implemented easily by individuals who did not have advanced scientific training. These shifts took the form of batches of product that differed significantly from other batches.

Arguably, the most influential contribution to measurement of health care quality occurred in the early 1960s when Donabedian[5] began to explicitly differentiate the quality measures related to structure, process, and outcome. The relative importance of process and outcome measures is still a subject of discussion in the contemporary literature, and Donabedian's general framework remains the dominant paradigm. Together, the three measures provide the best and most complete picture of quality.

In the last decade of the 20th century considerable efforts were made to implement approaches to quality measurement from industries outside of health care. One such approach is to apply measures of process and outcome to multiple domains of value across the organization. Kaplan and Norton[6] originally advocated this approach in the information technology industry. Batalden and Nelson[7] brought it to health care in the very practical form of scorecards and dashboards. Embedded in measurement tools is the understanding that the consideration of individual measures alone can be misleading, if not dangerous, because health care is a complex system subject to unintended consequences, and that multiple perspectives (e.g., patient, provider, payer) must be taken into account in the design of a useful measurement system.

## Types of Quality Measures

The gold standard for defining quality measurement remains Donabedian's three-element model of structure, process, and outcome.[8]

### Structural Measures

These relate to characteristics associated with a health care setting, including its design, policies, and procedures. The underlying assumption is that health care organizations that have the necessary quantity and quality of human and material resources and other structural supports are best prepared to deliver quality health care. Examples of structural measures include the availability of appropriate equipment and supplies in a hospital setting and the education, certification, and experience of clinicians in an institution.

Structure-focused measures often are easy to access. Health care organizations routinely maintain data on equipment and supply inventories, staffing, patient acuity, and staff qualifications. Unfortunately, adequate information on clinical processes often is difficult to obtain because most clinical databases lack sufficient process details.[9]

## Process Measures

*Process measures* evaluate if appropriate actions were taken for an intended outcome and how well these actions were performed to achieve a given outcome. The underlying clinical assumption is that if the right things are done right, the best patient outcomes are more likely to occur.[9,10] An example of an evidence-based process measure to assess the quality of care for a patient with acute myocardial infarction is the proportion of patients admitted with this diagnosis (without beta-blocker contraindications) who received beta-blockers within 24 hours after hospital arrival.

## Outcome Measures

*Outcome measures* seek to capture changes in the health status of patients following the provision of a set of health care processes and include the costs of delivering the processes. The patient is the primary focus, and outcome measures should describe the patient's condition, behavior, and response to or satisfaction with care. Outcomes traditionally are considered results that occur as a consequence of providing health care and cannot be measured until the episode of care is completed. Episodes of care may include hospitalizations, physician office visits, or care provided in postacute care settings. For example, to assess the quality of care for patients with acute myocardial infarction admitted to a coronary care unit, the outcome measures may be related to incidence of reinfarction and patient satisfaction with the care received in the unit.

Outcome measures provide an indirect measure of the overall quality of an organization and can provide trending and benchmarking opportunities to demonstrate progress. On the other hand, outcomes can be influenced by factors that are not measured or are beyond the control of clinicians, such as genomics, case mix, and socioeconomic or environmental influences. As a general rule, the more structure and process variables a QI project employs, the greater the reliability of outcome measures.[11]

Historically, quality measurement has focused primarily on outcomes. Today, structure and process measures provide important insights, illuminating which areas to address in order to improve outcomes. Structure and process provide direct measures of quality and thus yield more sensitive measures of quality, which can direct clinicians to the most effective ways to improve patient care. To be valid, however, structure and process must be empirically related to outcomes and be able to detect genuine differences in patient care. To maintain validity, they also must continually be reviewed and updated in accordance with current science (i.e., evidence).

## Constructing a Measurement

Comparisons of quality measures within systems and across providers require standards for how quality measures are expressed. The generally accepted standard for the expression of quality measures involves a numerator and a denominator. The numerator describes the desired characteristics of care, and the denominator specifies the eligible sample. For example, in the treatment of heart failure patients, the numerator for one possible proven measure is the number of people who actually receive beta-blockers, and the denominator is the number of people who are eligible to receive beta-blockers. Together, the numerator and denominator provide a measure of insight into the quality of the treatment of heart failure with beta-blockers.

Several factors should be considered when constructing a quality measure.[12] The age of the persons included, the measurement period, the system or unit being examined, and whether the measure will be within a program of care, across an entire health care setting, or local or national should be identified and considered.

The following strategies should be considered when constructing quality measures.

### Baseline Measurement

Almost all quality improvement processes, projects, or programs begin with the measurement of quality in its current state, which is known as a *baseline measurement*. Baseline measurements use many types of quantitative and qualitative data as indicators and allow a supporting analysis and an eventual judgment to be made about the status of medical quality at that point in time.

In Table 2-1, a baseline assessment is shown for a group of patients with diabetes whose hemoglobin (Hg) A1c levels were evaluated in year 1. This evaluation was used to design a QI project and to determine the change in HgA1c levels after 1 year of intervention.

The drawback to baseline measures is that they provide snapshots of measured characteristics of structure, process, or outcomes at one point in time. Measurement at another time can only be interpreted as higher or as lower than baseline and does not indicate actual or sustained improvement. Measurement tools that allow for trending are discussed in the next section.

### Trending Measurements

#### Run Chart

A *run chart* is a quality tool used to identify trends by measuring changes in structure, processes, or outcomes over time. The run chart is created in an XY graph in which the x-axis represents time, and the y-axis represents the aspect of the structure, process, or outcome being measured. A central line, if used, indicates the median of the data.

TABLE 2-1  Baseline Assessment: Hemoglobin A1c Levels at Baseline and After a One-Year Intervention for 212 Patients with Diabetes

**Member Interventions:**

☐  Applied program
— Stratification of diabetic population
— Special needs case management
— Outreach activities and education

☐  Referrals to employer program

**Provider Interventions:**

☐  Contacted physician and coordinated information

☐  Sponsored a physician education program

**Member Outcome:**

☐  Improved diabetes control
— Lowered hemoglobin A1c

**Direct Cost Savings:**

☐  Reduced hospital readmission rate for diabetes

|  | Hemoglobin A1c Levels | |
|---|---|---|
|  | Year 1 | Year 2 |
| N | 212 | 212 |
| Median | 7.30% | 7.10% |
| Average | 7.62% | 7.39% |
| % of Patients with Values <7.5% | 54.7% | 60.8% |
| % of Patients with Values >9.5% | 16.5% | 11.3% |

A *run* consists of consecutive points below or above the central line indicating a shift in the structure, process, or outcome measure being examined. A *trend* is a steady inclining or declining progression of data points representing a gradual change over time. Figure 2-1 provides an example of a run chart measuring length of stay over time. This run chart shows a decreasing trend in length of stay, which suggests that interventions targeting a reduction in length of stay may be effective, assuming average daily census and patient acuity have remained similar over time. Run charts provide ready information on runs and trends in structure, process, and outcomes and are easy to construct and interpret. For more statistical power, control charts are preferred.

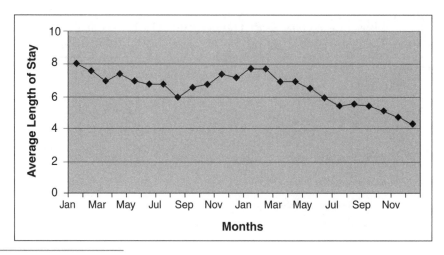

**Figure 2-1**  Example of a Run Chart for Average Length of Stay

## Control Chart

*Control charts* are most often used with process measures and are a more sensitive tool than run charts. The focus is not on trends but rather on process variation. Additional features include a central line composed of the mean value of the data and upper control limits (UCL) and lower control limits (LCL) typically representing three standard deviations from the mean.

A *statistical control chart* is a graph that represents the continuous application of a particular statistical decision rule to distinguish between normal and abnormal variations. Figure 2-2 shows a statistical control chart for the number of visits per day for a provider organization and covers each day during October 2008 (the PCL is the process control limit). The threshold is the point at which intensive evaluation or action is taken.

## Trigger Tools

One of the more promising areas emerging in quality measurement is the use of *trigger tools*. A trigger is an event that could potentially cause harm and is used to initiate further study.[13] The use of trigger tools affords a more rigorous opportunity to examine quality issues that have been traditionally based on less rigorous measures, such as self-report. Examples include certain drugs or abnormal lab values. For instance, orders for naloxone may signal a process error in pain management or sedation therapy.[14] Similarly, measuring the number of vitamin K administrations to patients receiving heparin may indicate process issues in anticoagulation therapy. The use of trigger tools expands the measurement of adverse events to include data on errors that do not result in harm. The approach adds substantial richness to data previously gathered because most errors do not result in injury.

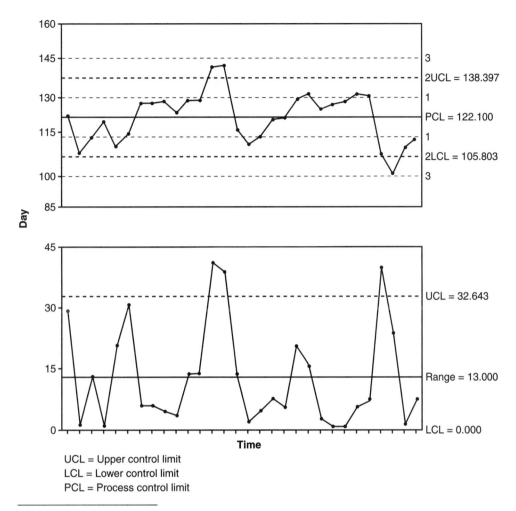

**Figure 2-2**   Example of Statistical Process Control Charts of Visits Per Day for a Physician Group

## Benchmarking

Quality improvement plans often include *benchmarking*, an effort to determine the current status of quality and compare it to the highest performers internal to an organization or external to the organization (e.g., comparing performance with competitors).[15]

An Achievable Benchmark of Care (ABC), as identified by Kiefe et al., is produced by benchmarks that (1) are measurable and attainable, (2) are based on the achievements of the highest performers, and (3) provide an appropriate number of cases for analysis.[16]

## CASE STUDY ● ● ●

### Cardiac Services, Dartmouth-Hitchcock Medical Center

The cardiac services unit at Dartmouth is one of the pioneers in contemporary approaches to measurement and improvement of health care quality. In their work,[17] measurement has been used as a central tool for tracking and improving care. They have argued persuasively that measurement of clinical process and outcome must be controlled by the clinicians delivering care. Several key principles defined their approach.

Clinicians were involved in the design of a panel of measures that were both useful to them in their daily practice and useful to administrators and external stakeholders. This panel encompassed the entire process of care and contained a balanced set of cost and quality measures. Patient-centered measures (e.g., satisfaction, functional status) were incorporated along with other traditional measures of process and outcome (e.g., mortality, morbidity). Details concerning variations were presented, as were aggregate measures over time. In addition, current variation was evaluated against historical performance using statistical process control charts.

Data for the project were obtained by chart abstraction in the perioperative period (i.e., at 3 weeks after surgery for satisfaction, at 6 months after surgery for functional status). Process variables were obtained in real time. The SF-36 indices of physical functioning, role functioning, bodily pain, and general health were used for the functional status measures. Among the measures of the surgical process were pump time, percent returning to pump, percent re-explored for bleeding, and internal mammary artery usage. Control charts were used with the surgical process data.

Control charts also were used for early detection of quality issues, allowing for near real-time correction. For example, the team was able to detect an increase in sternal wound infections by using a technique called a "successes between failures" chart to identify infrequent events and differentiate them from chance occurrences. This control chart allowed the team to decide if the increase in infections was due to random variation or a process shift. Because they used real-time data, they were able to quickly identify the process change related to this increase in infections and to correct it. Conventional methods usually result in delayed identification and more adverse events before solutions are found.

The results from this initiative are striking, although they cannot be attributed to measurement alone. Coronary artery bypass graft-related mortality dropped from 5.7% to 2.7% in a two-year period; the average total intubation time decreased from 22 hours to 14 hours; and the number of patients discharged in fewer than six days increased from 20% to 40%.

## Desirable Characteristics of Quality Measurement

Desirable characteristics for quality measures include relevance, meaningfulness or applicability, health importance or improvement, evidence-based, reliability or reproducibility, validity, and feasibility.[18]

## Relevance

The quality measure should be relevant to consumers, providers, clinicians, payers, and policy makers and should be of interest or value to the stakeholders and the project at hand.

## Evidence-Based

Quality measures, especially those related to clinical issues, should be based on sound scientific evidence. Measures should clearly link structure or process to outcomes.

## Reliability or Reproducibility

Reliability is the degree to which the quality measure is free from random error.[19] Measurement indicators and data collection techniques must be stable enough to justify the use of the collected information to make a judgment about quality. The same measurement process using the same data should produce the same results when repeated over time.

## Validity

Validity of a quality measure refers to the degree to which the measure is associated with what it purports to measure. A key question to be answered is whether the measures selected to indicate the presence or the absence of quality actually represent quality in patient care.

## Feasibility

Quality measures should be realistic and practical to collect and analyze. Measures that require too much time, money, or effort to collect may not be feasible to use.

# Interpreting Quality Measures

## Criterion-Based Measures

### *Appropriateness Model*

There are many ways to interpret quality measures. The Institute for Healthcare Improvement (IHI) advocates an "all-or-none" approach or *Appropriateness Model* to generate composite scores.[20] For example, if a patient with diabetes is expected to have a laboratory test, an eye exam, and a foot exam, failure to do any of these would result in failure of the composite measure of preventive diabetes care. The score reported reflects the proportion of patients who receive all of the care recommended for them.

The AHRQ uses the Appropriateness Model to arrive at composite scores and to produce a comprehensive overview of the quality of care delivered in the United States.

Composite measures based on this model are an increasingly large component of the report. AHRQ has chosen the Appropriateness Model because it reflects the philosophy that all citizens must receive all of the care that meets a high standard of evidence.

### The 70% Standard Model
A variation of this method sets the threshold at less than 100%, usually at 70% (the *70% Standard*). Although the all-or-none approach of the Appropriateness Model strives for perfection (and consequently results in lower scores than another method using the same dataset), this approach and the 70% Standard are sensitive to the number of indicators included in the composite.

## Opportunity Model

Another common approach is the *Opportunity Model* where the number of opportunities to deliver care is summed to create the denominator, and the number of cases in which indicated care is delivered is summed to create the numerator. The resulting percentage reflects the rate at which indicated care is delivered without penalizing some appropriate activities for the omission of others. This approach has been adopted by the CMS to reward hospitals for high performance (via pay-for-performance) in the Premier Hospital Quality Incentive Demonstration Project and internally in the Department of Veterans Affairs.

---

## CASE STUDY • • •
### *Fall Measurement at Baylor Health Care System*

Variables can often be measured in more than one way, and the method chosen should depend upon the audience and the intended use. The measurement of falls and falls with injuries provides a good example. Patient falls are often reported by prevalence or incidence per month, number of patients who fall divided by the total number of patients, and number of falls per 1000 patient days.

However, the *number of falls per month* lacks a reference point. An increase in the number of falls may be associated with an increased patient census, or it may be associated with more falls in a lower patient census. Hence, without a reference, it is difficult to interpret the simple expression of falls as a single number.

Measuring the number of patients who fall as a percentage of the total number of patients is another methodology. One can readily track the increase and the decrease in percentages, but it is difficult to benchmark internally or externally. One fall in a patient care unit of 10 patients is not the same as 1 fall in a unit of 30 patients. The former yields a percentage of 10% while the latter is 3.33%, and yet, the number of falls is the same.

Framing the measurement of falls by 1000 patient days allows for comparisons between hospitals of differing sizes and within units with variable patient census. It also allows for comparisons of frequency.

Managers, administrators, and quality improvement professionals typically track patient falls with one of the above methodologies, many reporting falls per 1000 patient days. Trending of these numbers over time allows for evaluation of improvement strategies. However, the above measurement methods provide insufficient feedback to frontline health care professionals, such as nurses, who are implementing strategies to decrease the number of patient falls.

A simple measure of falls used in patient care areas at Baylor is the number of days since the last fall. It is one number and easily understood—both the number and the goal it represents: to increasingly improve that number. While nurses cannot often tell you the number of falls on their unit per 1000 patient days or per total patients in a month, they can readily tell you the number of days since the last fall occurred. Baylor implemented this measurement on the front lines and found that people were better able to understand it, to speak it, and to use it to benchmark their own success.

The key is to make measurement usable. Match the user and the measure. If a measure is not useful, one should question why it is being measured.

## Program Evaluation

Program evaluation is necessary to measure the overall success of QI programs or projects and is usually conducted using two methods: formative evaluations and summative evaluations.

### Formative Evaluations

*Formative evaluations* involve routine examination of data on program activities and provide ongoing feedback about components of the program that work and those that require intervention. "Dashboards" and "scorecards" are tools used in formative evaluations to track and trend quality improvement activities on a monthly basis. They highlight key quality improvement initiatives and identify successful progress, thereby allowing for timely intervention as necessary. For example, the use of a dashboard for critical care may report monthly compliance with a ventilator-associated pneumonia bundle.

### Summative Evaluations

*Summative evaluations* are more formal and occur less often than formative evaluations, typically annually. Their focus is on measuring and determining the outcome or the effectiveness of the quality improvement program. The information evaluated is used to make decisions about the program, such as the need for more resources or education or perhaps better communication.

Effective program evaluations, whether formative or summative, are those that provide actionable information to program participants and management. Synthesis and use of information gleaned from program evaluations promotes the continuous development of the quality improvement program.

## Future Trends

We believe that quality measurement as a science will be the future.[21] A convergence of factors supports the need for increased rigor in quality measurement, including ongoing issues in the delivery of quality patient care, pay for performance, and growing consumer awareness. The desire to improve the rigor of measurement parallels the need to improve quality and safety in patient care. Timely acquisition and analysis of sound data through the increasing use of information systems and the use of reliable and valid measurement tools are essential. Rigorous quality measurement promotes the generalizability of findings in quality improvement initiatives, expanding their usefulness to the larger patient population.

CMS's pay-for-performance reimbursement strategy uses quality measurement to reward providers and practitioners for complying with evidence-based standards for providing patient care. By rewarding quality, the hope is that compliance with new efficacious treatments will increase and clinical outcomes will improve. Chapter 6 will provide more details on CMS's pay-for-performance strategies.

We believe that in addition to payers, consumers will drive improvements in quality measurement. Consumers are increasingly interested in health care delivery, especially as they assume greater responsibility for the cost of care, through increasingly higher premiums, deductibles, and co-pays.

Anything can be measured. How well something is measured is another issue. The challenge is to measure it well by focusing on the right structure, process, and outcome measures that are relevant, meaningful, important, evidence based, reliable, valid, and feasible.

## References

1.  Scobie S, Thomson R, McNeil J, Philips PA. Measurement of the safety and quality of health care. *MJA.* 2006;184(suppl 10):S51–S55.
2.  Codman EA. The end result idea and the product of a hospital: A commentary. *Arch Pathol Lab Med.* 1990;114(11):1105.
3.  Donabedian A. The end results of health care: Ernest Codman's contribution to quality assessment and beyond. *Milbank Qtrly.* 1989;67(2):233–256.
4.  Shewart W. *Economic Control of Quality of Manufactured Product.* New York: D. Van Nostrand Company, Inc.; 1931. (Republished in 1981 by American Society for Quality.)
5.  Donabedian A. *Explorations in Quality Assessment and Monitoring. Vol 1: The Definition of Quality and Approaches to Its Assessment.* Chicago, IL: Health Administration Press; 1980.
6.  Kaplan RS, Norton DP. *The Balanced Scorecard: Translating Strategy into Action.* Boston: Harvard Business School Press; 1996.
7.  Nelson EC, Mohr JJ, Batalden PB, Plume SK. Improving health care, part 1: The Clinical Value Compass. *Jt Comm J Qual Improv.* 1996;22(4):243–258.
8.  Donabedian A. Evaluating the quality of medical care. *Milbank Qrtly.* 1966;44:166–206.
9.  Palmer RH. Process-based measures of quality: The need for detailed clinical data in large health care databases. *Ann Int Med.* 1997;127(8 Pt2):733–738.
10. Ranson SB, Maulik SJ, Nash DB. *The Healthcare Quality Book: Vision, Strategy and Tools.* Chicago, IL: Health Administration Press; 2005.

11. Mant J. Process versus outcome indicators in the assessment of quality in health care. *Intl J Qual Health Care*. 2001;13(6):475–480.

12. Agency for Healthcare Research and Quality. Evaluation of the AHRQ QI Program. http://www.ahrq.gov/about/evaluations/qualityindicators/qualindch4.htm. Accessed September 30, 2007.

13. Resar RK, Rozich JD, Classen D. Methodology and rationale for the measurement of harm with trigger tools. *Qual Saf Health Care*. 2003;12(suppl 2):39–45.

14. Rozich JD, Haraden DR, Classen D. Adverse drug event trigger tool: A practical methodology for measuring medication related harm. *Qual Saf Health Care*. 2003;12:194–200.

15. Mohr JJ, Mahoney CC, Nelso ED, Batalden PB, Plume SK. Improving health care, part 3: Clinical benchmarking for best patient care. *Jt Com J Qual Improv*. 1996;22(9):599–616.

16. Kiefe CI, Weissman NW, Allison JJ, et al. Identifying achievable benchmarks of care: Concepts and methodology. *Int J Qual Health Care*. 1998;10(5):443–447.

17. Nugent WC, Schultz WC, Plume SK, et al. Design an instrument panel to monitor and improve coronary artery bypass grafting. *JCOM*. 1994;1(2):57–64.

18. Institute of Medicine, Committee on the National Quality Report on Health Care Delivery. *Envisioning the National Health Care Quality Report*. Washington, DC: National Academies Press; 2001.

19. National Quality Measures Clearinghouse. Glossary. http://www.qualitymeasures.ahrq.gov/resources/glossary.aspx. Accessed October 14, 2007.

20. Nolan T, Berwick DM. All-or-none measurement raises the bar on performance. *JAMA*. 2006;295(10):1168–1170.

21. Harrington L, White S. Interview with a quality leader: Mark Chassin, new president of the Joint Commission. *J Healthc Qual*. 2008;30(1):25–29.

Chapter 3

# Patient Safety

*Philip J. Fracica, MD, MBA, FACP, Sharon Wilson, RN, BS, PMP, and Lakshmi P. Chelluri, MD, MPH, CMQ*

## Executive Summary

Accidents inevitably occur—people in all lines of work make errors. The Institute of Medicine (IOM) report *To Err Is Human*[1] brought to the forefront the issue of medical errors and the resulting risks to patient safety and preventable adverse events. Recognition that high-reliability organizations (HROs) such as aviation and the nuclear power industry improved safety by focusing on organizational processes led to a closer examination of organizational issues in health care. Today, there is more of a focus to create a transparent culture that addresses safety from an organizational perspective.

There are a number of tools, systems, methodologies, resources, and patient safety products to help guide the implementation of safe practices. Analytic tools can provide powerful insights into the causes of a poor outcome. Understanding the causes of errors and failures are important; using that understanding to change the process is critical to improvement. Designing systems that make it difficult for people to make mistakes and easy for them to do the right thing is often referred to as "hard wiring" for reduced risk.

There are several general strategies that consistently improve the safety and reliability of processes, including those listed below (to be discussed in detail in this chapter):

- Reduced reliance on memory with automation, algorithms, and easily accessible references.
- Simplification through reduction of unnecessary process steps and hand-offs.
- Standardization to reduce variation.
- Use of constraints to eliminate undesired behavior and forcing functions to assure desired behavior.
- Careful and appropriate use of protocols and checklists.
- Improved access to information at the point of care.
- Reduced reliance on vigilance through automation, alarms, and scheduled monitoring.
- Cautious use of automation to avoid introduction of new errors, to avoid staff complacency, and to maintain individual responsibility.

*Learning Objectives*

Upon completion of this chapter, readers should be able to:

- describe the history and development of patient safety initiatives;
- discuss a systems approach to the prevention of errors;
- describe the different types of errors that pose risks to patient safety;
- identify issues in organizational culture than can affect error reporting;
- describe processes to identify and analyze errors; and
- explain how teamwork and crew resource management can improve patient safety.

# History

From the time of Hippocrates, the primary goal of medicine has been to improve the health of individuals, or at least to "do no harm." In the 19th century, physicians recognized that infections could be acquired at the hospital, and Semmelweis[2] proposed hand washing prior to patient contact to decrease puerperal fever. Unfortunately, 150 years after Semmelweis's proposal, hand washing is still not universal. In the early 20th century, Codman[3] listed errors due to deficiencies in technical knowledge, surgical judgment–diagnostic skills, and equipment as causes for unsuccessful treatments. Schimmel[4] studied adverse events in a group of hospitalized patients in 1964 and reported that 20% of patients admitted to medical wards suffered an adverse event and that 6.6% of the adverse events were fatal. Since Schimmel's initial report, there have been multiple studies[5] reporting an adverse event rate of 2% to 4% of hospital admissions.

In 1994, Leape[5] brought a new perspective on errors in medicine by focusing on the psychology of error and human performance, arguing that fundamental change would be needed to reduce errors. Media attention to high-profile adverse events cases raised awareness of safety issues in the health care system, prompting the landmark IOM report on medical errors and patient safety.

Anesthesia is the epitome of success in patient safety efforts to reduce medical errors. The field's focus on detecting adverse events and prevention of harm has led to the decrease in the number of anesthesia-related deaths from 3.7/10,000 anesthetics to 1 to 2/200,000 in ASA I or II patients,[6] reaching the levels achieved by HROs such as aviation.

In the past decade, there has been increased focus on improving patient safety. Although significant progress has been made since the publication of the IOM report, Altman[7] in 2004 reported that 50% of the public was concerned with the safety of health care and 40% believed that the quality of heath care actually had gotten worse.

# Error as a Systems Issue

Systematic studies of organizational accidents have led to an understanding that errors do not occur as isolated events but are shaped by the nature of the organization in which they occur. This insight has led to deeper understanding of how organizations can act as complex adaptive systems and how system factors can contribute to errors. The metaphor of a sword or spear has been used to describe the dichotomy between the work itself and the processes that support that work, with the term "sharp end" serving as a label for the direct action elements of work and "blunt end" serving as a convenient term for the support functions of work.

Unsafe acts can be direct hazards or can act to weaken existing defenses. These errors, referred to as *active failures*, occur at the sharp end. When accidents occur, active failures are often relatively easily identified, and blame is commonly assigned to one or more individuals at the sharp end. This focus on the sharp end has been described as the "person approach" because it emphasizes assigning blame to individuals. A problem with this approach is that active failures are virtually never intentional and are usually not random occurrences.

Errors tend to fall into recurrent patterns. A focus on individual culpability for error can divert attention away from a "systems approach" to uncover the cause of the error. Active failures of individuals are often symptoms of overlooked, deeper *latent conditions*. Examples of latent conditions include poor supervision and training; poor design of work tasks; inadequate staffing levels; impractical and unworkable processes; inadequate tools; and poorly designed and implemented automated systems. Each of these latent conditions can weaken the barriers that protect patients from harm. The latent conditions can be thought of as scattered holes in the barriers so that the layers of defense are more like a series of slices of Swiss cheese[8] (Figure 3-1).

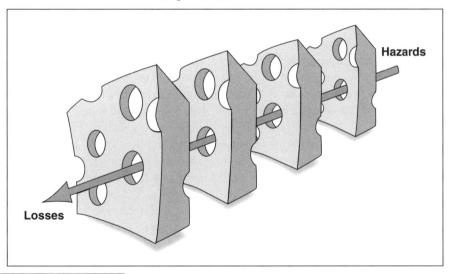

**Figure 3-1**   The *Swiss Cheese* Model of Hazards, Defenses, Barriers, and Accident Trajectories That Produce Harm

*Source:* Reason J. The human error. BMJ. 2000;320:768–770.

Latent conditions are represented by existing holes in layers. Active failures can be represented as new holes that are created. Harm results when an occasional hazard travels along a "golden trajectory" along which the holes in the slices all line up, allowing the hazard to make its way through all the safeguards and result in an accident. This is a useful conceptual model because it makes it easy to see how both the frequency of the hazards and the number and the adequacy of the layers of defense will interact to produce an accident. It is well accepted that most accidents occur when an unlikely combination of multiple failures, each insignificant alone, combine to create the necessary circumstances to allow a disaster to occur.

There are many levels that contribute to the health care system, and each can provide a frame of reference within which to identify latent factors that can contribute to patient harm (Table 3-1).

Study of active failures[9] reveals that the majority do not occur due to negligence or disregard. Most health care errors are made by individuals who are competent and well motivated. Active failure can be viewed as failure to achieve a desired outcome that occurs when the wrong plan is selected or when the right plan is poorly executed. Active failures can be classified as failures of three common types of activities: skill-based, rule-based, and knowledge-based activity.

*Skill-based* activity is characterized by a familiar task, performed by an experienced individual. It is rapid, automatic, effortless, and requires little conscious feedback. Obtaining and recording vital signs, dispensing medication, and stocking supplies by experienced individuals are examples of health care skill-based activities. Active failures of skill-based activities can also be described as *failures of execution*. The individual intends to perform the correct activity but unconsciously deviates from the intended task. Anyone who has planned to make an unfamiliar stop on the trip home from work only to proceed directly home has personally experienced a skill-based activity failure. Slips, lapses, omissions, duplications, and confusion are examples of active failures of skill-based activity. Routine and habit are important contributors to these errors. When attention wavers, individuals will naturally revert to a familiar habit.

*Rule-based* activity can be accomplished by breaking the task up into a group of "if–then" rules. *Mistakes* are errors that involve a wrong intention or plan and are the cause of active failures of rule- and knowledge-based activities. The wrong plan may be selected because a bad rule is being used, a good rule is being misapplied, or other relevant rules are being ignored.

Often complex processes, such as the development of a diagnostic and therapeutic plan, are reduced to the application of appropriate rules and result in mistakes based on rule-based activity failure. For example, the use of routine empiric therapy for community-acquired pneumonia for a patient with significant immune compromise would represent a rule-based mistake. As medical knowledge advances and more protocols and algorithms are validated, many knowledge-based activities have and will become

**TABLE 3-1  Framework of Factors Influencing Clinical Practice and Contributing to Adverse Events**

| Framework | Contributory Factors | Examples of Problems That Contribute to Errors |
|---|---|---|
| Institutional | • Regulatory context<br>• Medicolegal environment | Insufficient priority given by regulators to safety issues; legal pressures against open discussion, preventing the opportunity to learn from adverse events |
| Organization and management | • Financial resources and constraints<br>• Policy standards and goals<br>• Safety culture and priorities | Lack of awareness of safety issues on the part of senior management; policies leading to inadequate staffing levels |
| Work environment | • Staffing levels and mix of skills<br>• Patterns in workload and shift<br>• Design, availability, and maintenance of equipment<br>• Administrative and managerial support | Heavy workloads, leading to fatigue; limited access to essential equipment; inadequate administrative support, leading to reduced time with patients |
| Team | • Verbal communication<br>• Written communication<br>• Supervision and willingness to seek help<br>• Team leadership | Poor supervision of junior staff, poor communication among different professions; unwillingness of junior staff to seek assistance |
| Individual staff member | • Knowledge and skills<br>• Motivation and attitude<br>• Physical and mental health | Lack of knowledge or experience; long-term fatigue and stress |
| Task | • Availability and use of protocols<br>• Availability and accuracy of test results | Unavailability of test results or delay in obtaining them; lack of clear protocols and guidelines |
| Patient | • Complexity and seriousness of condition<br>• Language and communication<br>• Personality and social factors | Distress; language barriers between patients and caregivers |

*Source:* Vincent C. Understanding and responding to adverse events. *NEJM.* 2003; 348:1051–1056. © 2003 Massachusetts Medical Society. All rights reserved.

rule-based activities. Computerized "expert systems" that apply intricate systems of inter-acting rules and algorithms to manage difficult clinical situations may further blur the distinction between rule-based and knowledge-based activities in the future.

*Knowledge-based* activity occurs with a novel task. It tends to be slower, requiring con-scious thought, mental effort, and awareness. Knowledge-based activities are those where the intended outcome cannot be achieved by the mere application of rules. Failure to establish the correct diagnosis and therapy in a challenging case is an example of the failure of a knowledge-based activity.

## Human Factors as a Cause of Errors

Inherent limitations to human performance, referred to as *human factors*, contribute to the occurrence of errors. Understanding human factors is essential to effectively identifying the root causes of errors and to facilitate the design of systems that are error resistant. Strategies to reduce failures of skill-based activity include work flow design that reduces interruption and distractions, the use of checklists, conscious pauses, forcing functions, and automation. Human factors are important determinants of skill-based errors and also influence more complex knowledge-based problem-solving activities. For example, consider confirmation bias, the tendency to favor solutions that have been initially iden-tified in lieu of potentially better solutions and to selectively filter data to reinforce a chosen course. Once a physician arrives at a tentative diagnosis (even if incorrect), there is a tendency to emphasize information that supports the diagnosis and to minimize con-flicting data. In order to avoid confirmation bias, it is better for two individuals to inde-pendently make a calculation or observation and then to compare results than for one individual to "check" the result of another.

### Fatigue

Although traditionally physicians have worked prolonged hours, the impact of sleep deprivation on medical errors has received more attention after the death of Libby Zion.[10,11]

---

## CASE STUDY • • •

### *Death of Libby Zion*

Libby Zion was an 18-year-old woman admitted to a New York hospital with fever and agita-tion, who died within 24 hours. Her father, journalist Sidney Zion, suggested that inadequate supervision of house staff, high workload, and long hours led to errors in her care that resulted in her death. As a result of this incident, the Bell Commission was formed to review the prac-tices and suggest changes. Although the commission reported that both supervision and work hours were a concern, the issue of work hours received more publicity. As a result, the state of New York mandated changes in resident work hours in 1989. The limitation on work hours was adopted by the Accreditation Council on Graduate Medical Education (ACGME) in 2003.

These changes were controversial within the medical profession for a number of reasons: the need for increased hand-offs, which itself could cause additional errors; the lack of convincing data to support the perception that longer shifts adversely impact patient care; and the concern about loss of professionalism. However, most training programs voluntarily implemented the changes due to the threat of losing accreditation and the possibility of government legislation.

---

Health care workers are exposed to multiple factors that put them at increased risk for developing fatigue. These include nonstandard schedules (shift work and night shifts), interaction with and responsibility for acutely ill patients, need for continuous vigilance, work-related stress and physical fatigue, and inadequate rest and sleep.

Sleep loss and disruption of circadian rhythm is shown to affect performance; Dawson[12] reported that the performance of an individual without sleep for 24 hours is similar to one with an alcohol level of 0.1%. Sleep loss and fatigue can result in depression, anger, anxiety, irritability, and decreased psychomotor function. Sleep loss results in nanonaps, where the individual falls asleep for a few seconds at a time without realizing it. These brief lapses increase the potential to make an error.

Shift work increases the risk of fatigue because of inadequate rest between shifts and decreased ability of the body to adjust to changes in shift between day and night. The two most vulnerable periods of the day are mid-afternoon (around 3 p.m.) and early morning (around 3 a.m.), and nursing shifts longer than 12 hours and work weeks longer than 40 hours are risk factors for fatigue and increased errors.[13-15] The effects of fatigue become cumulative if the rest periods are inadequate, resulting in development of chronic fatigue. Multiple interventions have been implemented in the past few years to address fatigue in health care workers, particularly among physicians in training. The interventions include limiting the number of duty hours and altering schedules to allow for adequate rest between on-call hours, providing nap periods during the shift, using stimulants, avoiding double shifts for nurses, providing bright lighting, helping with development of healthy sleep habits, standardizing processes, and simplifying tasks. More study is needed regarding the effectiveness of interventions to decrease fatigue and medical errors.

## Medication Errors

Modern pharmacologic agents are potent modulators of physiologic processes. If used optimally, these actions can produce significant improvements in patient morbidity and mortality; however, failures of the medication system can produce significant harm. A *medication error* is any error occurring in the medication use process. To clearly understand the patient safety implications of the medication system, it is important to define some important relevant terms.

An *adverse drug event* (ADE) is an unexpected or dangerous reaction to medication. Some adverse drug events are the result of medication errors and have also been referred to as *preventable adverse drug events*. Due to individual variability, it is impossible to accurately predict the consequences of the use of any medication—for example, allergic reactions in patients not known to have drug sensitivity and idiosyncratic drug reactions.[16] The term *adverse drug reaction* is synonymous with nonpreventable adverse drug event.

Medication errors can be categorized by the process that has failed.[17]

*Prescribing errors* involve the assessment of the patient, clinical decision making, drug choice, dosing interval and duration of therapy, documentation of the decision, and generation of an order or prescription. Although prescribing is the responsibility of the physician or nonphysician advanced practitioner, prescribing errors can result from system problems such as failure to provide relevant information about previously identified drug allergies. Prescribing errors may include failure to prescribe beneficial therapy, prescription of an ineffective medication, failure to dose appropriately, failure to consider interactions with other medications and foods, comorbid medical conditions, and significance of known hypersensitivity. Prescribing errors can also occur due to poor documentation or communication of the drug order. Illegibility and the use of potentially ambiguous abbreviations are common causes of medication error at the prescribing step. Prescribing errors may be identified by pharmacy staff, nursing staff, or other members of the care team, and interventions can be taken to avert an adverse event.

*Transcription errors* occur in the hospital environment when the physician's medication order in the patient chart is incorporated into the Medication Administration Record used to manage and document the administration process. Transcription errors can occur when a written physician order is incorrectly transcribed into the pharmacy record system. The transcription process usually involves communication of the written medication order to the pharmacy. Communication of the order can occur through physical delivery of a copy of the order by courier or pneumatic tube system or through electronic communication through use of telephone, fax, or digital scanning technology. Once received, the order is transcribed into the pharmacy information system and incorporated into the Medication Administration Record provided to nursing staff. A transcribing error may represent a failure in both prescribing and transcribing. The generation of an unclear drug order is the prescribing error, and the failure to identify or to clarify the ambiguous order represents a transcribing error. The risk of transcription error is even higher when the initial order is verbal or provided by telephone.

*Dispensing errors* include errors related to medication mixing or formulation, transfer of medication from stock supply to patient containers, double-checking, labeling, and other documentation. The dispensing process is usually performed by pharmacy staff. In the hospital environment, dispensing errors occur when the pharmacy staff dispenses drugs that differ in some way from the transcribed order. Outpatient dispensing errors occur when the medication dispensed differs from the written prescription. Dispensing orders may result due to confusion over drugs that may have similar names or appearance (look-alike and sound-alike medications).

*Administration errors* involve the actual introduction of the drug in the patient. The drug may be administered by nursing staff or other caregivers or may be self-administered by the patient. Administration usually includes verification of the order or instructions, preparation or measuring of the dose, and actual administration via the proper route in the proper fashion. Administration errors include omitted doses, duplicated doses, incorrect time of administration, administration of medications that were not ordered, administration of incorrect quantity, and administration by an incorrect route. Drugs administered by intravenous infusion carry the additional risk of inappropriate infusion rate.

*Monitoring errors* involve the assessment of the intended therapeutic effect and the identification of unintended adverse consequences. The monitoring may be done by the patient or by health care professionals. In either case, feedback must be provided to the prescribing practitioner and documented so that the therapy can be optimized. Monitoring errors include failure to recognize that the expected benefit has not occurred and failure to identify drug-induced adverse effects. The incidence of medication errors is as noted in Table 3-2.

## Measurement of Medication Errors

It has been difficult to arrive at authoritative determination of the prevalence and significance of medication errors and ADEs. Wide variation in measurements can occur depending upon the type of methods used to detect and record these occurrences. Staff may be encouraged to self-report medication errors using manual reporting forms or incident reports. Direct observation of drug administration, with comparison with the written physician order, provides very accurate and much higher measurements of medication error rates. The direct observation method is often impractical, as it is resource intensive and dependent upon the availability of trained observers.

There is similar variation in reporting of ADEs. Self-reporting by staff produces relatively low rates. Review of randomly chosen hospital medical records by expert reviewers

---

### TABLE 3-2 Incidence and Responsibility for Medication Errors

| Subprocess | Frequency (Bates*) | Physician | Pharmacy | Nurse |
|---|---|---|---|---|
| Prescribing | 56% | +++ | + | +/− |
| Transcribing | 6% | + | +++ | − |
| Dispensing | 4% | − | +++ | − |
| Administration | 34% | − | − | +++ |

*Bates' frequency data adapted from:* Leape LL, Bates DW, Cullen DJ, et al. Systems analysis of adverse drug events: ADE Prevention Study Group. JAMA. 1995;274:35–43. Reprinted with permission from the Journal of the American Medical Association.

trained to identify adverse drug events generally produces the highest measured rates; however, the resources required for chart extraction limits the extent to which this method is employed. The use of trigger tools[18] to prescreen charts for exhaustive review has been shown to be effective and efficient. This method is described in detail in Chapter 2.

The most common medication errors occur in prescribing and medication administration. Prescribing error incidences of 15 to 1400 errors per 1000 hospital admissions have been reported. Prescribing errors can also be recorded in terms of errors per 1000 orders, with a range of 0.5 to 50 errors per 1000 hospital medication orders. Administration errors are the most common, with reported incidences ranging from 3% to 11% of doses. Considering the number of medication doses that patients typically receive during a hospital admission, it is apparent that most hospitalized patients are likely to experience one or more medication errors over the course of their stay. Medication administration errors in nursing home populations have been found to be about twice as frequent as the hospital inpatient rates.[19]

Fortunately, many medication errors do not result in measurable harm to patients. The reported incidences for preventable ADEs range from 1 to 2 events per 100 hospital admissions or 3 to 6 events per 1000 patient days. Medication errors account for between 25% and 50% of all ADEs in the inpatient setting, excluding patients in nursing homes. Ordering errors and administration errors are consistently the most frequent causes of preventable ADEs, collectively accounting for about three-quarters of the total.[19]

Information failures, including lack of knowledge about the drugs and lack of information about the patients, are a major system cause of medication errors.

### Strategies to Prevent Medication Errors

**Effective Systems Interventions**    The routine *inclusion of an indication* for the drug order is an important safeguard against order misinterpretation. This practice can prevent pharmacy staff from misinterpreting a poorly legible drug name. It can also help pharmacy staff to recognize when a physician has confused two drugs and ordered the wrong one through a slip, a lapse, or poor knowledge about the medication. Providing an indication could conceivably have the unintended consequence of additional physician calls when drug use for an off-label indication is misinterpreted as an ordering error. As safeguards become more robust, the chances increase that legitimate interventions will be intercepted or delayed. The appropriate "tuning" of safeguards to optimize safety without undue compromise of efficiency is likely to remain a major challenge for the foreseeable future.

Particular caution in the labeling, the storing, and the handling of drugs that either look alike or sound alike can also help prevent mix-ups throughout the entire process. Labeling of drugs with "tall man" lettering, which emphasizes the differences between similar sounding drugs, is a useful safety intervention to reduce dispensing errors.

The development of standardized drug formulary lists reduces the number of medications used in a health care organization. This standardization makes it easier for staff to become familiar with the available drugs, making everyone involved in the transcription of orders or the dispensing of drugs less prone to error. The potential benefits of a standardized formulary can be further leveraged through the use of standardized medication management protocols and order sets (e.g., weight-based heparin protocols or standardized insulin protocols). However, there are potential safety issues that must be addressed when discharging patients whose medication was switched in case the formularies of the ambulatory drug plan are different or a generic is used that is a different color or shape.

The use of standardized concentrations for intravenous infusions can reduce errors in dispensing and administration.[19] Similarly, *computerized physician order entry* (CPOE) can reduce errors in the ordering phase and eliminate transcribing errors because the physician order is directly entered into the pharmacy information system. As powerful as many of the individual safeguards are, they provide even greater benefit when used together.

**Medication Reconciliation**  *Medication reconciliation* is a process that enables the review and documentation of the most complete and accurate list of medications a patient is taking. Accurate medication reconciliation can help prevent ordering errors of omission, may uncover likely drug–drug interactions (herbal and over-the-counter medications), and may prevent duplication of medications. The availability of relevant patient-specific information and drug information (such as age, renal and hepatic function) as the order is being written can also prevent errors. Poor legibility or the use of error-prone abbreviations are common sources of error in the ordering phase.

**Computerized Physician Order Entry**  *CPOE* allows practitioners to generate medication orders or prescriptions through a computer system. (More details are available in Chapter 5, Informatics.) In addition to addressing problems of legibility and miscommunication, the automated system contains relevant patient data and may generate real-time alerts to the practitioner as the order is being written. Although CPOE holds promise for reducing or eliminating many current errors,[19] this technology represents a major redesign of a complex process and, as such, may well introduce new failure modes as it reduces or eliminates specific known errors. Potential problems with CPOE systems include the difficulty in appropriately tuning the sensitivity of the alerts. If alerts are generated even when there is a low risk of an order causing harm, then the system will have a high sensitivity (miss very few ordering errors) but will have a poor specificity (generate many false alarms). If too many alerts are generated, practitioners will become conditioned to ignore or override the alerts.

**Automated Pharmacy Systems**  Automated systems similar to CPOE are currently used by pharmacists during the transcription or dispensing phases. The pharmacist notifies the physician when a potential ordering error has been detected. A central part of the dispensing process involves the physical movement of the drug from a storage area into a packaging designed for administration. For outpatient medications, dispensing may involve counting out pills from a large container into a pill bottle containing several days' supply. For hospital patients, it may involve placing the proper medications into a drawer in a medication cart or the dispensing may be done by an automated drug dispensing unit on the inpatient unit (which must be periodically correctly restocked by the pharmacy). For intravenously administered medications, the mixing of the drug infusion is a critical part of the dispensing process. The use of premixed solutions and standardization of the concentration of infused drugs help reduce errors.

The development of automated robotic devices to dispense medication from pharmacy stocks and automated equipment to formulate complex infusion mixtures are revolutionizing dispensing. Some of the more advanced robotic dispensing systems include motorized robotic transport carts carrying drugs to resupply automated dispensing units. An important requirement for automated dispensing systems is an ability to label individual drug doses in a manner that can be easily recognized by the system, such as optical bar coding. Because pharmaceutical manufacturers have failed to incorporate standardized bar code identification into their drug packaging, additional automated equipment is required to repackage unit doses of drugs with bar-code identifiers to facilitate automation of the medication administration system.

**Redundancy for Safety**   The administration process is the source of a relatively large number of medication errors, which are difficult to intercept or detect. These errors can include administration of the wrong drug or wrong dose at the wrong time as well as the omission or duplication of scheduled doses. Patients may be misidentified and receive medications intended for other patients. Some high-risk medications are routinely double-checked by a second nurse before administration. However, this type of safeguard is particularly vulnerable to the slips and lapses that humans inevitably manifest, because the double-checking process requires prolonged attention and concentration.

**Forcing Functions**   The design of technology to prevent unsafe modes of operation is referred to as *forcing functions*. A good example of this method of risk reduction is infusion technology. Drugs administered by intravenous infusion carry additional risks. If the drug is infused too rapidly, an overdose will occur. Errors in calculating infusion rates from drug concentration are well described, particularly with drugs dosed by patient weight. Because infusion pumps remain continuously at the bedside, errors have occurred when patients inadvertently alter the pump settings. Safeguards against infusion pump medication administration errors include limitations of the amount of drug contained within the reservoir and the incorporation of safety features into the design of infusion pumps. Standard infusion pump safety features include "no free-flow" design and locking mechanisms to prevent unauthorized tampering. Newer safety features include smart pump technology. Smart pumps contain microprocessors programmed with upper dose limits for infused drugs. When the infusion is attached to the pump, the nurse is required to indicate the drug and the concentration. If the pump is set for an infusion rate greater than the upper safety limit for that drug, an alert will be triggered, and the pump will not deliver the excessive rate.

**Patient Empowerment**   Patients and their families can provide an important safeguard at the medication administration phase by asking questions about any medication they are receiving and the reason it is being given. They should also be encouraged to fully disclose all medications, supplements, and over-the-counter medications. Patient involvement can be particularly helpful to safeguard against allergies and inadvertent omission of chronic maintenance medications, which should not be interrupted.

## Common Risks to Patient Safety

### Invasive Procedures

Surgical and other invasive procedures have many risks. Many of the risks are influenced by the specialized skills of the operator or the procedure team and are inherently difficult to safeguard against with generic risk-reduction strategies.

Some general risk factors apply across a wide range of *invasive procedures*. One of the most basic safety factors involves verification to prevent wrong site surgery. This process ensures that the correct patient is about to undergo the correct procedure on the correct site and that the correct equipment (including implants) is available. The use of a preprocedure "pause" to complete a checklist to verify each of these elements is an important safety step. Best practice is to have a well-developed script that the surgeon, anesthesiologist, and nurse all utilize. These improvements are based on the aviation model of crew resource management[20] and can help reduce errors in the hierarchical operating room environment.

Patient management by anesthesiologists is generally highly standardized and includes some of the most robust safety engineering found in health care.[6] Many minor invasive procedures involve minimal or moderate sedation and local anesthesia and do not routinely require the presence of an anesthesia specialist. Over-sedation during procedures or during postprocedure recovery can lead to respiratory compromise. The use of sedation protocols and postprocedure care protocols developed in collaboration with anesthesia specialists can help reduce this risk.

Some operative procedures require prophylactic antibiotic administration that must be timed to coincide with the surgical incision to optimally protect against wound infection. Standardized processes for incorporating the antibiotic administration into the operating room work flow help avoid errors of omission. Other safety risks associated with surgical procedures include the risk of retained surgical equipment and the risk of transfusion reaction if blood delivered to the operating room is brought to the wrong patient. For invasive procedures such as thoracocentesis, paracentesis, organ biopsies, and central venous catheter insertion, the use of diagnostic imaging such as ultrasonography can help reduce complications.

Fire safety is also important in the operating room and other procedural areas where oxygen, combustible materials, and energy sources such as high-intensity illumination, lasers, and cautery devices are combined.

## Infections

Hospital-acquired infections (HAI) have received increased attention due to their overwhelming consequences in terms of cost, morbidity, and mortality. CMS and other payers have begun to refuse reimbursement for additional care resulting from treatment for an infection not present on admission.[21] Consistent, mindful adherence to basic infection control principles, usually referred to as *universal precautions*, is a critical protective strategy that too often fails. These measures include hand decontamination upon entering and leaving every patient encounter. The use of alcohol-based skin cleansers is highly effective and convenient. For patients with certain particularly dangerous types of infections, isolation and the use of disposable gowns and gloves in addition to hand decontamination can help limit patient-to-patient spread. It is important to remember that any physical objects, such as pens, documents, or medical equipment, that come into contact with the patient can also transmit infections and should be decontaminated or sequestered. Close attention to maintenance of normal range blood glucose levels has been shown to be an effective intervention to reduce the incidence of multiple types of HAIs.

### Site-Specific Infection Prevention

**Postoperative Surgical Wound Infections**     Appropriate surgical site preparation through the use of hair clippers rather than shavers and the use of chlorhexidine-based cleansing agents has been shown to be important.[22-25] The appropriate timing and selection of prophylactic antibiotic therapy also reduces infections.

**Ventilator-Associated Pneumonia**     Important interventions shown to reduce the incidence of ventilator-associated pneumonia include minimizing the duration of intubation; maintaining effective oral hygiene; elevating the head of the bed by at least 30°; minimizing opening of the ventilator circuit; avoiding prolonged uninterrupted sedation; and using endotracheal tube designs, which allow continuous removal of subglottic secretions.

**Central Venous Catheter Infections**     Effective interventions to decrease the incidence of central venous catheter infections include the use of chlorhexidine-based skin cleansers; the use of sterile technique and full barrier precautions; the selection of the subclavian insertion site over femoral or internal jugular sites; the use of chlorhexidine-containing insertion site dressing; and the use of antimicrobial bonded catheter technology.[26]

**Urinary Tract Infection**    Avoidance of unnecessary or prolonged use of indwelling bladder catheters is the most important method of reducing urinary infections.

**Resistant Organisms**    The emergence of virulent pathogens, which are resistant to multiple antimicrobial agents, is a major threat. Specific organisms of concern include methicillin-resistant *Staphylococcus aureus* (MRSA), vancomycin-resistant enterococcus (VRE), gram negative organisms producing the extended-spectrum beta-lactamase (ESBL) resistance factor, and other multiple drug resistant strains of gram negative infections such as pseudomonas and acinetobacter. Because patients can be asymptomatic carriers of resistant organisms, some health care organizations are employing active surveillance procedures in which cultures are routinely obtained at scheduled intervals to promote earlier identification of resistant organisms. Beyond isolation measures, the careful management of antibiotic use is an important intervention to limit the development of these types of infections. It is important to carefully manage antimicrobial formularies and to implement mechanisms to monitor and to control the appropriate use of selected antibiotics that promote the development of resistance. Close cooperation among medical staff, infection control, pharmacy, and clinical microbiology professionals is essential for the development of effective institutional control measures.

## Patient Falls

*Falls*, with resultant injury, represent a significant risk for adverse patient outcomes. Unfortunately, some falls result in serious injuries such as hip fracture, subdural hematoma, or intracranial hemorrhage. One of the best general prevention strategies is effective assessment in order to recognize patients at risk for falls.[27] Risk factors intrinsic to the patient include altered mental status, reduced vision, musculoskeletal disease, history of previous falls, and presence of acute and chronic illness. Extrinsic risk factors are those present in the patient's environment and include sedating medications, elevated beds, absence of grab rails, ill-fitting footwear, poor illumination, unstable flooring, and inadequate assistive devices. Once the risk has been identified, appropriate patient-specific measures should be implemented to reduce the risk. These can include modifications to the patient's environment, patient education, and adequate assistance and supervision, in some cases including the use of sitters.

## Pressure (Decubitus) Ulcers

*Pressure ulcers* occur when tissue is compressed between bony prominences and external surfaces for sufficient duration to cause tissue necrosis. Ulcers commonly occur in soft tissue overlying the sacrum, ischial tuberosities, thoracic spine, and heels. Pressure ulcers may require extensive surgical interventions and can lead to systemic infection, sepsis, and death. Due to the serious sequelae, prevention, early diagnosis, and interventions are key management strategies. Common risk factors include immobility, inactivity, nutritional compromise, fecal and urinary incontinence, and impaired ability to perceive or to respond to sensations of soft tissue discomfort.

Several validated risk assessment tools have been developed (e.g., the Braden Scale, Norton Scale, and Gosnell Scale).[28-30] It is important that patients be adequately assessed for the risk of ulcer development, as well as the actual presence of ulcers. Preventive strategies include optimization of skin care, pressure reduction through use of cushioning, and frequent repositioning. In patients at risk for pressure ulcers, particular care must be taken to avoid friction injury or abrasion during repositioning. Reversible causes of fecal and urinary incontinence should be evaluated and treated. If the incontinence cannot be prevented, absorbent materials designed to transfer moisture away from the skin surface should be used. Continued education of health professionals, patients, and families is also an important preventive strategy.[31]

## Patient Safety Tools

### Tools for Data Acquisition

#### Safety Surveys

Safety culture assessment tools are used for developing and evaluating safety improvement interventions in health care organizations and provide a metric by which the implicit shared understandings about the expectation of how things are done are made available. A number of national organizations (e.g., the Leapfrog Group, the National Quality Forum [NQF], the American Medical Association, and the American Hospital Association) have designed or promote various survey tools. One of the most commonly used hospital surveys is the AHRQ's Hospital Survey on Patient Safety Culture.[32] A key advantage of using these tools is that national sharing of data can provide local and national benchmarks for comparison. Similar culture surveys have been customized to address specific populations or health care settings, such as surgical areas of a hospital, nursing homes, nurses, and nursing assistants.

#### Error Reporting

The reporting of errors or unexpected negative events provides a critical data source. Every error that is recognized and examined provides an opportunity to learn how the system can avoid repeating it. Classification of events into various categories can help organizations keep track of events and determine what type of action plan is appropriate. *Preventable adverse events* are acts of omission or commission resulting in harm to the patient. *Close calls* or *near misses* are events or situations that could have resulted in an adverse event but did not. *Sentinel events* are unexpected occurrences involving death, serious physical or psychological injury, or risk thereof, and can be considered to be the subset of adverse events containing the most serious occurrences. The reporting of such events, either through a mandatory or voluntary reporting system, provides critical data necessary to understand the risk and motivate effective action to reduce the risk.[33]

Incident reporting is a common formalized method of reporting the actions of oneself or others in the health care environment.[34] Such systems may use simple paper forms with check boxes and areas for recording event characteristics or more sophisticated networked computer-based applications that interface directly into data systems. Incident reporting is an important means of capturing information on errors and adverse events. Some states[34] have established formal incident reporting structures, which allow statewide benchmarking.

In organizations with a punitive culture, staff may be reluctant to generate reports that could create negative consequences for themselves or colleagues. For this reason, incident reporting systems are likely to underestimate actual numbers of incidents. Underreporting makes it difficult to establish clear benchmarks and standards of practice, because reports are influenced both by the frequency of occurrence of events and by the willingness of staff to report those events. As a result, organizations that are likely becoming safer may observe an increase in reported events as they develop systems to reduce risk.

### Self-Reporting Systems

*Self-reporting systems*, a subset of incident reporting, are often unique to an individual organization or an organizational system. The intent is to gather and aggregate data that can be used to create safety alerts and tips, to identify and showcase best practices, and to highlight trends. Self-reporting systems that are unique to an organization lack an in-depth common language that can hinder learning and minimize comparative data for benchmarking.

### Record Review

*Record review* has long been used as a primary tool for a morbidity and mortality committee to identify contributory factors, which indicate areas for improvement and prevention. Gathering information helps to develop a collective picture of a practice that can identify the outlier or unusual event during a particular procedure/process. Targeted record reviews aimed at sentinel events, high-rate incidences, or other trigger events yield important epidemiological information. Screening charts for the presence of several markers for adverse events can be used to trigger a more thorough review of the records. For example, the administration of the drug naloxone, which reverses or antagonizes the effects of opiate analgesic agents, can be considered a marker for opiate overmedication. A review of 20 charts of patients who received naloxone is likely to yield a much higher incidence of opiate overmedication than a random sample of 20 charts. The Institute for Healthcare Improvement (IHI) has developed a standardized trigger tool to identify records that are more likely to contain adverse events or errors.[18]

The increasing use of electronic medical records offers the potential for an automated review of records for the presence of triggers. This is particularly exciting because it can address attention to a case while the patient is still being actively treated during the same care encounter. When a patient is noted to have a pattern suggestive of an adverse event, a timely focused review may help to identify the problem and to avert a negative outcome.

## CASE STUDY • • •

### An Innovative Event Recognition System

Many institutions utilize Medical Emergency Teams (MET) (also known as Rapid Response Teams [RRT]) to manage acute patient decompensation. The University of Pittsburgh Medical Center (UPMC) has used feedback from MET interventions to detect medical errors.[35] UPMC initiated a review of MET responses performed by a group led by senior medical staff and administration in order to identify medical errors and address the cause of errors. Approximately one-third of the MET responses involved errors (both diagnostic as well as treatment errors). The information from MET reviews is provided to the unit managers and staff for review and suggestions for improvement. The proposed changes to address identified issues are presented at the hospital-wide Patient Safety Committee meeting for approval. The MET reviews resulted in interventions to decrease misplacement of feeding tubes, improve management of hyperglycemia resulting in better glycemic control, and decrease in hypoglycemic episodes.[36–38] The medical director and nursing leadership provide support and coordinate implementation of interventions with individual departments.

*Situation monitoring* of error events, also known as *direct observation*, is the process of actively scanning and assessing routine health care standards of practice delivery (e.g., hand washing or medication administration). Monitoring situational elements provides understanding of event error in real time and helps to maintain functional awareness of practices. Observation of clinical events performed by different practitioners can also lead to the development of more standardized approaches to care.

Increasing emphasis is being placed on required reporting. In *To Err Is Human*, the IOM called for a nationwide mandatory reporting system that would provide for the collection of standardized information about adverse events that result in death or serious harm.[1] To date, there is no national reporting requirement. All states license hospitals and require them to comply with specific requirements to ensure that minimum health, safety, and quality standards are maintained. As of 2002, 20 states had enacted mandatory reporting of adverse events as part of health care facility state licensure requirements.

Proponents of *public reporting* believe it will help accelerate the pace of improvement throughout the health care industry and provide individuals with the information needed to make informed decisions about their own care and to protect themselves against adverse medical events. Those who are concerned about public reporting claim that it may result in physicians refusing to care for high-risk patients. The use of data for internal performance improvement and the safe practice of medicine is supported by all.

## Analytic Tools

### Retrospective Event Analysis

Critical or sentinel events have been identified as particularly concerning. Most organizations have processes for performing a rigorous detailed analysis of such events in order to prevent recurrence. A prerequisite to solving and eliminating a problem is finding the root cause. *Critical event analysis* or *root cause analysis* (RCA) is a practical problem-solving tool used to define the problem, to identify the cause(s) (often at multiple levels), and to create solutions.

The tools used as part of the RCA process can be grouped into several categories: data collection, event understanding, possible cause analysis, cause and effect, and pattern recognition. Reliable data is an essential foundation for a successful RCA; data collection supports and substantiates analysis. Flow charts (Figure 3-2) are important tools that are used to recreate the problem or event to gain understanding.

Brainstorming is used to generate multiple ideas, which are then evaluated to reach consensus over the significance of these possible causes as a contributing factor to the event. Scoring mechanisms can provide a more structured framework to determine the relative importance of the potential causes identified through brainstorming. The U.S.

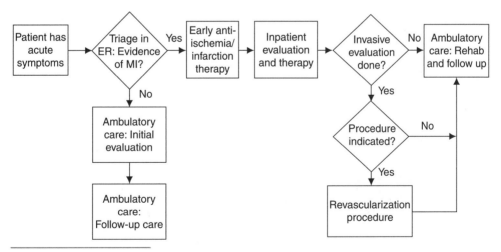

**Figure 3-2**  Sample High-Level Flow Chart: Ischemic Heart Disease Patient Flow (IHI Tool)

*Source:* Reprinted with permission of the Institute for Healthcare Improvement (http://www.IHI.org).

Department of Veterans Affairs (VA) *Safety Assessment Code* (SAC) matrix, developed by the VA in partnership with AHRQ and the National Center for Patient Safety, is an easy-to-use method for analyzing the key factors of severity and probability of adverse events and near misses or close calls.[39]

## Pareto Charts

*Pareto charts* (Figure 3-3) can help to identify dominant causes among the possibilities when quantitative data exist as to the frequency of the various causes. Visual diagrams help identify patterns, dominant causes, relationships between two causes, or other variables. *Histograms* and *scatter* or *affinity charts* (Figure 3-4) can help identify these patterns.

## Fishbone Diagrams

Fishbone diagrams (Figure 3-5) are another important RCA tool, invented by Dr. Kaoru Ishikawa, to determine the root causes in an event. The fishbone provides a systematic way of looking at the effects and the causes that create or contribute to those effects. Other methods to facilitate cause-and-effect analysis include *matrix diagramming* (to arrange

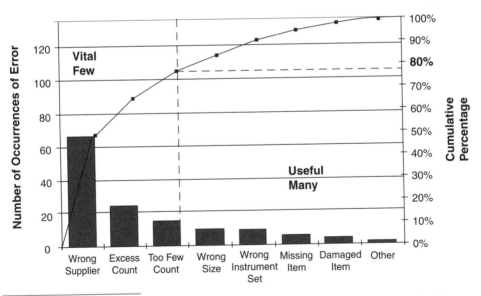

**Figure 3-3** Sample Pareto Diagram: Types of Errors Discovered During Surgical Setup (IHI Tool)

*Source:* Reprinted with permission of the Institute for Healthcare Improvement (http://www.IHI.org).

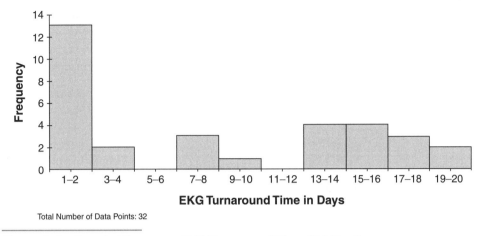

**Figure 3-4**   Sample Histogram: EKG Turnaround Time (IHI Tool)

*Source:* Reprinted with permission of the Institute for Healthcare Improvement (http://www.IHI.org).

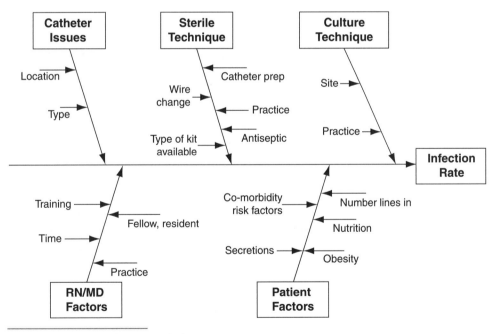

**Figure 3-5**   Root Cause Analysis

*Source:* Frankel H, Crede W, Topal S, Roumanis M. Use of corporate six sigma performance: RCA of catheter-related bloodstream infections in a surgical ICU. *J Am Coll Surg.* 2005:201(13):349–358. Reprinted with permission from Elsevier.

pieces of information according to certain aspects) and the "Five Whys" (used in brainstorming to delve more deeply into causal relationships). The latter method involves asking the question "why?" in reference to the initial event and repeating it again four more times in response to each answer. Each repetition of the question can uncover a deeper level of contributing causes.

### Prospective Event Analysis

#### Failure Mode and Effects Analysis (FMEA)

FMEA was developed as an engineering design tool for the aerospace industry in the mid-1960s, specifically looking at safety issues; it has since become a key tool for improving safety in many industries, including health care. FMEA is a systematic method of identifying potential failures, effects, and risks within a process with the intent of preventing problems before they occur. This requires careful analysis of the current process at a fairly detailed level, using input from individuals who are experienced in the day-to-day practical operations.

Each way that the process can fail is a failure mode. Each potential failure mode has a potential effect with an associated relative risk. The relative risk of a failure and its effect is determined by three factors: severity (the consequence of the failure); occurrence (the probability or frequency of the particular mode of failure); and detection (the probability of the failure being detected before harm occurs). By multiplying the severity, occurrence, and severity subscores, a composite risk profile number (RPN) can be determined for each potential failure mode. This method allows calculation of an overall process risk score and allows prioritization of the relative importance of any particular step in the overall process. Finally, it allows an organization to model the reduction in overall risk as changes in high-risk elements of the process are implemented. (This tool may also be referred to as a *proactive risk assessment.*)

## Disclosure of Errors

The increased focus on errors and their disclosure to patients and families has a profound impact on health care workers (HCWs). Successful strategies to address the impact on house staff include accepting responsibility, constructive changes in practice, advice about avoiding recurrence, and provision of emotional support.[39,40]

HCWs—physicians in particular—are reluctant to discuss errors with patients and families or peers for a variety of reasons: difficulty in defining errors; complex emotional reactions (anger, guilt, shame, embarrassment); sense of autonomy and individual responsibility; loss of self-esteem; concern about perception of peers and patients; perceived lack of feedback and support from the organization; and concerns over financial and legal liability. The disclosure of error is sometimes partial or misleading because of the perceived uncertainty about the relationship between the error, the harm, and the natural progression of the disease.

Interviews with patients and families reveal a concern about lack of disclosure of errors. Patients and families suggest that describing the mistake (explaining what happened), apology, steps to minimize recurrence, and compensation, when appropriate, would address the issue of disclosure. In spite of the HCW concerns about family–patient perception, surveys show that disclosure could improve the relationship with patients.[34,41-44] Reports of disclosure programs, implemented by the University of Michigan and the VA hospital in Lexington, did not show an increase in malpractice costs.[44,45] The impact of widespread use of these programs on litigation and malpractice is not clear.

# Prevention of Errors

## Systems Approach

Leaders play a large role in creating and nurturing the *culture of safety* that is an essential requirement for high-reliability health care organizations.[46] By partnering with staff, health care leadership can create a workplace environment that minimizes latent factors, which help to generate errors. A culture of safety challenges leaders to look beyond assigning blame to an individual and instead to address underlying system problems.

Organizations with a positive safety culture are characterized by communications founded on mutual trust, by shared perceptions of the importance of safety, and by confidence in the efficacy of preventive measures. Key measurements of safety performance should be systematically recorded, monitored, and openly discussed so that the organization can track progressive improvements in safety.

In a culture of safety, the reporting of errors and near misses is rewarded and viewed as an important contribution that helps identify and improve unreliable processes. The use of nonpunitive reporting policies for self-reported errors helps encourage open communication about latent conditions. Individuals are accountable not only to successfully accomplish tasks but to identify and report failures and to identify conditions that promote failure. Standardized rituals that help promote safety can be incorporated into routine clinical unit work flow to create opportunities for staff to consider and to discuss potential safety problems. Patients should be empowered with knowledge and information so that they can participate in their own care and support efforts designed to safeguard them from harm.

Health care leaders should become familiar with the topic of patient safety and frequently discuss the subject in communications with staff, physicians, patients, the public, and organization governing board members. Members of the senior administrative team should periodically visit frontline staff (in patient care areas and in support services) to discuss safety concerns and conduct.

Leaders should promote organizational transparency and openness. Formal disclosure policies can help reinforce the message of transparency and openness about errors. The free flow of information that comes with openness and transparency also helps build *learning organizations*.[47] Learning organizations that are continually growing and improving incorporate information from internal and external sources.

## CASE STUDY ● ● ●

### Culture of Safety

Sentara Health system, a 6-hospital integrated health care system in southeastern Virginia, achieved a 46% reduction in the incidence of serious adverse events after implementing a systemwide patient safety initiative. The commitment of senior leadership was key to the program's success. Key components included integration of patient safety concerns into the development of strategic priorities, staff incentives, human resource policies, and resource allocation. Fifty percent of the organization's employee incentive gain-sharing program was based on safety and quality measures. Both hospital staff and medical staff were involved in the process. Operational leaders were given responsibility for implementing the program.

The program utilized training in behavior-based expectations. All staff members were expected to demonstrate the following: Pay Attention to Detail, Communicate Clearly, Have a Questioning Attitude, Hand off Effectively, and Never Leave Your Wingman. Organization leaders were expected to demonstrate accountability, to promote safety, and to provide continuous reinforcement of the commitment to safety. Medical staff were to utilize physician-to-physician communication for consultations and to clearly designate a physician responsible for coordinating the care for each individual patient.

## Operational Interventions to Prevent Error

An understanding of the human factors that lead to active failures can help health care organizations design resilient systems that provide safeguards against slips, lapses, and mistakes. *Forcing functions* are an important protection against slips in action. Forcing functions constrain behavior by either forcing individuals to consciously consider a suspect action or even by making certain types of actions impossible. Computer alert messages that require positive confirmation before files are deleted or potentially dangerous files are accessed are examples of forcing functions.

Forcing functions that provide warnings or alerts that must be addressed can be easily incorporated into automated systems; however, they must be used judiciously. Excessive use of some forcing functions can actually increase the risk of errors. If staff members are continuously faced with a stream of cautions concerning very low-risk possibilities, the alerts will gradually become ignored. The use of aids such as checklists, redundant double checking, reminders, and automated prompting systems all help prevent skill-based slips and lapses. The use of information technology to automate repetitive skill-based tasks is likely to be an increasingly important innovation to reduce error. It is likely that we will see revolutionary redesign in health care work flow processes in the near future as networked information technology devices become smaller and move out to the point of care.

## CASE STUDY • • •

### *Forcing Functions*

Improper positions of central venous catheters can result in positioning the catheter tip within the right atrium. This presents a risk of catheter erosion through the thin atrial wall with resulting potentially lethal cardiac tamponade. After observing two cases of fatal cardiac tamponade due to this problem in their hospitals, the Los Angeles County Department of Health Services identified that a significant percentage of central venous catheters in their facilities were being advanced too far. They identified evidence in the medical literature that identified a reduced risk of this problem if 16 cm length catheters were used. The standard catheter length for their facilities was changed from 20 cm to 16 cm, resolving the problem with the catheter malpositioning. The switch to the shorter catheters was a forcing function, which prevented the problem of overinsertion. An added, and unforeseen, benefit was a significant reduction in the number—and the cost—of repeat chest radiographs that had been used to adjust the position of the longer catheters.

## Decision Support Systems

Health care organizations need to function under extreme variations of activity and stress. Emergency departments are subject to particularly chaotic swings in activity and acuity due to the open access to the community and the rapid turnover time for patients. Within minutes, emergency departments can transition from being almost empty with no serious cases to large numbers of patients waiting to be seen, while the staff tries to manage several simultaneous life-threatening conditions. Health care organizations can define various operating states that require different types of support and resources. When certain threshold triggering conditions are met, the organization can implement standardized preconceived contingency plans. This strategy can be employed by clinical units that might transition between condition green, condition yellow, and condition red, with each operating state triggering different levels of staffing, resources, and operating procedures. This creates a safer, more reliable system by turning the problem of what to do under peak demand conditions from a knowledge-based task where solutions are worked out "on the fly" to a rule-based task. The activation of specialized response teams to deal with high-risk events such as cardiac arrest and major trauma is another example of how health care organizations can dynamically reorient resources to effectively meet emergent needs.

Reduction in variation through the use of standardized protocols and order sets can be a powerful strategy to reduce errors. As information system technology becomes more sophisticated, more complex rules will likely be developed. These sets of complex rules have been referred to as *decision support systems*, and they offer the promise of combining the benefits of standardized rules while avoiding the risk of oversimplification of complex situations.

## Teamwork and Crew Resource Management

Missed communication and miscommunication are the most common causes of sentinel events analyzed by the Joint Commission.[48] Teamwork provides a defense against error by individuals by providing monitoring and double checking. *Crew Resource Management* (CRM),[20,49-51] a tool used in aviation to improve safety, focuses on how human factors interact with stressful environments. The components of CRM are situational awareness, problem identification, decision making, workload distribution, time management, and conflict resolution. The goals of CRM are error avoidance, prevention of progression of an error, and mitigating the harm from the error. Team training provides a shared understanding of the task and goals and improves communication between team members with differing expertise.

In the past few years, there has been an increased emphasis on adopting the CRM principles to medical settings. CRM or Medical Team Training (MTT) programs for emergency medicine, operating room, and intensive care unit (ICU) staff have been introduced to improve communication and teamwork.[49,52] Although CRM training is reported to change attitudes in medical settings, more studies are needed on the appropriate format for implementing CRM principles and the impact on adverse events. STEPPS (Strategies & Tools to Enhance Performance & Patient Safety) is another multicomponent program, designed by the U.S. Department of Defense, that aims to improve teamwork through mutual support, leadership, situation monitoring, and communication.[53]

An approach that has been successfully used to improve communication in teams and access providers is to standardize the format for communication between staff and physicians through use of the SBAR tool:[54]

- **S**–situation: description of clinical situation
- **B**–background: clinical history and context
- **A**–assessment: a description of the possible problems
- **R**–recommendation: a description of possible solutions

It is also critically important to effectively communicate at points of "hand-offs" or transitions in care. As the responsibility for the patient is transferred from one individual to another, there is a heightened risk that disruptions will occur. This risk can be mitigated by organizing work flow to minimize the frequency of transition and through the development of effective hand-off communication.

## High-Reliability Organizations (HROs)

HROs[55] are routinely exposed to unexpected high-risk events, yet they are able to achieve lower than expected occurrences of failure or accidents. Classic examples of HROs include air traffic and electrical power grid control systems, nuclear power plants, and aircraft carriers. Diverse types of HROs display certain common cultural attributes and institutional capabilities.

*Preoccupation with failure* is an important attribute of HROs. This involves constant vigilance and a commitment to compulsively and rigorously focus on any and all failures, large or small, regardless of whether actual harm occurred. This vigilance can be manifested by an organization's ability to identify and report errors, to investigate errors, and to implement effective measures to prevent recurrence. Poor outcomes rarely occur without warning; in the vast majority of cases, the root causes that ultimately led to disaster were known within the organization but tolerated because they were unlikely to cause "real problems."

Ironically, organizations with very high standards for success and performance may be culturally incompatible with a preoccupation with failure. The temptation of the organization that values high performance is to view individuals who display a concern over small failures as "nay sayers" who are standing in the way of success. Senior leaders may create a "shoot the messenger" culture where they end up being buffered from the reality of what is going on in the organization. Preoccupation with failure also implies a measurement culture that continuously monitors key processes and includes feedback mechanisms to identify and to correct deficiencies. When errors are identified, they should be investigated to identify the human active failures and the latent system conditions that contributed to the error.

A *reluctance to simplify* is another characteristic of HROs, which are commonly very good at simplifying complexity in order to maintain a focus on areas of high priority and key performance drivers. Unfortunately, complex interactive systems are not easily reduced to simple rules. Oversimplification generates operational practices that may work very well in most cases but fail spectacularly when the uncommon complication occurs. Organizations that resist simplification are less likely to experience these types of adverse events.

HROs also demonstrate *sensitivity to operations*. The latent conditions that create the "Swiss cheese holes" in system safeguards are frequently well known to those at the organization's sharp end. To the extent that managers are removed from day-to-day operations, or even worse, actively discourage feedback from frontline staff, these latent conditions may go uncorrected. HROs have organizational cultures that (1) promote understanding of frontline operational issues and open communication of operations problems throughout the organization and (2) are committed to correcting operational problems as they are discovered.

*Deference to expertise*, another attribute of HROs, can be viewed as a part of sensitivity to operations. Deference to expertise refers to the practice of pushing decisions down to the level of the individual most knowledgeable about the process involved, regardless of their position of authority within the organizational hierarchy. A practical example would be involving clerical staff in a redesign of a patient scheduling process.

HROs also share the quality of *resilience*, which refers to the ability of an organization to effectively respond to unanticipated threats and to recover from disruptive events. Standardized, well-thought-out policies and procedures generally promote safety. However, HROs can recognize when hazards that occur are not being successfully addressed by existing procedures. The ability to identify and to adapt to novel situations and crises is a critical attribute of HROs. This requires an ability to optimize standardization while maintaining an ability to respond to challenges that require new solutions. This has been referred to as "constrained innovation" or "adaptive rule-breaking."

## Future Trends

We believe that the topic of patient safety will become an increasingly important and critical focus of the health care industry for the foreseeable future. We expect to see increasing focus on the elimination of error and adverse events and full disclosure of errors to patients and the health care system.

In addition to increasing scrutiny and transparency of event reporting, there will likely be an increase in insurers' refusals to pay for care resulting from adverse events and complications. CMS has already begun to withhold payment for specific conditions that were not documented to be present on admission.

There will likely be increasing incentives for the health care system to eliminate adverse events. Traditional expectations that certain complications should be considered expected or unavoidable will likely be increasingly challenged. We are already seeing coordinated programs to reduce risk, which are demonstrating dramatic improvements in nosocomial catheter-related and ventilator-associated infections.

The proliferation of electronic medical records and the availability of bedside "smart devices" will hopefully improve documentation and reduce opportunities for human error. We predict that automation is likely to proliferate particularly for repetitive operations requiring concentration and vigilance, which humans do not do well. The use of robotic systems for dispensing and labeling drugs and bedside barcode scanning to assist in medication administration are notable examples.

## References

1. Institute of Medicine. *To Err Is Human: Quality Chasm Series.* Washington, DC: National Academies Press; 1999.
2. Nuland SB. *The Doctors' Plague: Germs, Childbed Fever, and the Strange Story of Ignac.* New York/London: W.W. Norton & Co.; 2003.
3. Mallon WJ. *Ernest Amory Codman. The End Result of a Life in Medicine.* Philadelphia, PA: W.B. Saunders; 2000.
4. Schimmel EM. The hazards of hospitalization. *Qual Saf Health Care.* 2003;12:58–64. (Reprinted from *Ann Intern Med.* 1964;60:100–110.)
5. Leape LL. Error in medicine. *JAMA.* 1994;272:1851–1857.
6. Pierce EC Jr. The 34th Rovenstine lecture. 40 years behind the mask: Safety revisited. *Anesthesiology.* 1996;84:965–975.
7. Altman DE, Clancy C, Blendon RJ. Improving patient safety: Five years after the IOM report. *N Engl J Med.* 2004;351:2041–2043.
8. Reason J. The human error. *Brit Med J.* 2000;320:768–770.
9. Vincent C. Understanding and responding to adverse events. *N Engl J Med.* 2003;348: 1051–1056.

10. Lerner BH. A case that shook medicine. How one man's rage over his daughter's death sped reform of doctor training. *Washington Post*. November 28, 2006. http://www.washington post.com/wp-dyn/content/article/2006/11/24/AR2006112400985_pf.html. Accessed December 28, 2007.

11. Asch D, Parker R. The Libby Zion case: One step forward or two steps backward? *N Engl J Med*. 1988;318:771–775.

12. Dawson D, Reid K. Fatigue, alcohol, and performance impairment. *Nature*. 1997;388:235.

13. Gaba DM, Howard SK. Fatigue among clinicians and safety of patients. *N Engl J Med*. 2002;347:1249–1255.

14. Parshuram CS. The impact of fatigue on patient safety. *Pediatr Clin N Am*. 2006;53:1135–1153.

15. Steinbrook R. The debate over residents' work hours. *N Engl J Med*. 2002;347:1296–1302.

16. Leape LL, Bates DW, Cullen DJ, et al. Systems analysis of adverse drug events. *JAMA*. 1995;274:35–43.

17. Bates DW, Cullen DJ, Laird N, et al. Incidence of adverse drug events and potential adverse drug events. Implications for prevention. ADE Prevention Study Group. *JAMA*. 1995;274:29–34.

18. Rozich JD, Haraden CR, Resar RK. Adverse drug event trigger tool: A practical methodology for measuring medication related harm. *Qual Saf Health Care*. 2003;12:194–200.

19. Board on Health Care Services. *Preventing Medication Errors: Quality Chasm Series*, 1st ed. Washington, DC: National Academies Press; 2007.

20. Healy GB, Barker J, Madonna G. Error reduction through team leadership: Applying aviation's CRM model in the OR. *Bull Amer Coll Surg*. 2006;91:10–15.

21. FY 2008 inpatient prospective payment system final rule. Improving the quality of hospital care. Centers for Medicare and Medicaid Services Website http://www.cms.hhs.gov/apps/media/press/factsheet.asp?Counter=2338. Accessed July 1, 2008.

22. Ko W, Lazenby WD, Zelano JA, et al. Effects of shaving methods and intraoperative irrigation on suppurative mediastinitis after bypass operations. *Ann Thorac Surg*. 1992; 53(2):301–305.

23. Balthazar ER, Colt JD, Nichols RL. Preoperative hair removal: A random prospective study of shaving versus clipping. *South Med J*. 1982;75(7):799–801.

24. Horgan MA, Piatt JH Jr. Shaving of the scalp may increase the rate of infection in CSF shunt surgery. *Pediatr Neurosurg*. 1997;26(4):180–184.

25. Fletcher N, Sofianos D, Berkes MB, et al. Current concepts review: Prevention of perioperative infection. *J Bone Joint Surg*. 2007;89:1605–1618.

26. Veenstra DL, Saint S, Saha S, Lumley T, Sullivan SD. Efficacy of antiseptic-impregnated central venous catheters in preventing catheter-related bloodstream infection: A metaanalysis. *JAMA*. 1999;281:261–267.

27. American Geriatrics Society, British Geriatrics Society, American Academy of Orthopaedic Surgeons Panel on Falls Prevention. Guideline for the prevention of falls in older persons. *J Am Geriatr Assoc*. 2001;49(5):664–672.

28. Bergstrom N, Braden BJ, Laguzza A, Holman V. The Braden Scale for predicting pressure sore risk. *Nurs Res*. 1987;36(4):205–210.

29. Hodge J, Mounter J, Gardner G, Rowley G. Clinical trial of the Norton Scale in acute care settings. *Aust J Adv Nurs*. 1990;8(1):39–46. [Norton scale for decubitus prevention.] *Krankenpflege (Frankf)*. 1980;34(1):16.

30. Gosnell DJ. Pressure sore risk assessment: A critique. Part I. The Gosnell scale. *Decubitus*. 1989;2(3):32–38.

31. Maklebust J, Sieggreen M. *Pressure Ulcers: Guidelines for Prevention and Nursing Management*. 3rd ed. Springhouse, PA: Springhouse; 2001.

32. U.S. Department of Health and Human Services, Agency for Healthcare Research and Quality. Hospital Survey Form. http://www.ahrq.gov/qual/hospculture/hformtxt.htm. Accessed October 1, 2008.

33. Wald H, Shojania KG. Incident reporting. In: *Making Health Care Safer: A Critical Analysis of Patient Safety Practices*. Evidence Report/Technology Assessment No. 43, AHRQ Publication No. 01-E058; July 2001. http://www.ncbi.nlm.nih.gov/books/bv.fcgi?rid=hstat1.section.59490. Accessed January 25, 2008.

34. Leape LL. Reporting of adverse events. *NEJM*. 2002;347:1633–1638.

35. Braithwaite RS, DeVita MA, Mahidhara R, et al. Use of medical emergency team (MET) responses to detect medical errors. *Qual Saf Health Care*. 2004;13:255–259.

36. Mardrstein EL, Simmons RL, Ochoa JB. Patient safety: Effect of institutional protocols on adverse events related to feeding tube placement in critically ill. *J Am Coll Surg*. 2004;199:39–47.

37. Dinardo MM, Naschese M, Korytkowski M, Freeman S. The medical emergency team and rapid response system: Finding, treating, and preventing hypoglycemia. *Jt Comm J Qual Saf*. 2006;32:591–595.

38. Donihi AC, Dinardo MM, Devita MA, Korytkowski MT. Use of a standardized protocol to decrease medication errors and adverse events related to sliding scale insulin. *Qual Saf Health Care*. 2006;15:89–91.

39. U.S. Department of Veterans Affairs. National Center for Patient Safety. *Safety Assessment Code (SAC) Matrix*. http://www.va.gov/ncps/SafetyTopics/HFMEA/HFMEA_SAC.html. Accessed July 1, 2008.

40. Wu AW, Folkman S, McPhee SJ, et al. Do house officers learn from their mistakes? *JAMA*. 1991;265:2089–2094.

41. Gallagher RM, Levinson W. Disclosing harmful medical errors to patients: A time for professional action. *Arch Int Med*. 2005;165:1819–1824.

42. Gallagher TH, Waterman AD, Ebers AG, et al. Patient and physician attitudes regarding disclosure of medical errors. *JAMA*. 2003;289:1001–1007.

43. Witman AB, Park DM Hardin SB. How do patients want physicians to handle mistakes? A survey of internal medicine patients in an academic setting. *Arch Intern Med*. 1996;156:2565–2569.

44. Gallagher TH, Studdert D, Levinson W. Disclosing harmful medical errors to patients. *N Engl J Med*. 2007;356:2713–2719.

45. Kraman SS, Hamm G. Risk management: Honesty may be the best policy. *Ann Intern Med*. 1999;131:963–967.

46. Reason J. *Managing the Risks of Organizational Accidents*. 1st ed. Burlington, VT: Ashgate Publishing Company; 1997.

47. Senge P. *The Fifth Discipline: The Art & Practice of the Learning Organization*. New York: Doubleday; 2006.

48. Anonymous. Poor communication is common cause of errors; communication critical, says JCAHO official. *Health Care Benchmarks and Quality Improvement* (BNET Business Network); August 2002. http://findarticles.com/p/articles/mi_m0NUZ/is_/ai_90683346. Accessed October 1, 2008.

49. Grogan EL, Stiles RA, France DJ, et al. The impact of aviation-based teamwork training on the attitudes of health-care professionals. *J Am College of Surgeons*. 2004;199:843–848.

50. Oriol MD. Crew resource management. Applications in healthcare organizations. *J Nurs Adm*. 2006;36:402–406.

51. Dunn EJ, Mills PD, Neiely J, et al. Medical team training: applying crew resource management in the Veterans Health Administration. *Jt Comm J Qual Patient Saf.* 2007;33:317–325.
52. Department of Defense. *About Team STEPPS™: DoD Patient Safety Program.* http://dodpatientsafety.usuhs.mil/teamstepps. Accessed March 19, 2008.
53. Leonard M, Graham S, Bonacum D. The human factor: The critical importance of effective teamwork and communication in providing safe care. *Qual Saf Health Care.* 2004;13(suppl 1): i85–i90.
54. Weick KE, Sutcliffe KM. *Managing the Unexpected: Resilient Performance in an Age of Uncertainty.* 2nd ed. San Francisco: Jossey-Bass; 2007.
55. Agency for Healthcare Research and Quality. High reliability organizations: Organizational advice. http://www.ahrq.gov/qual/hroadvice. Accessed October 9, 2008.

## Additional Resources–Further Reading

The Joint Commission (TJC; http://www.jointcommission.org) provides assistance in the form of requirements for accredited health care organizations including annual National Patient Safety Goals.

The Institute for Safe Medication Practices (ISMP; http://www.ismp.org) is an excellent resource for information about safety in the medication system and pharmacy practice.

The Institute for Healthcare Improvement (IHI; http://www.ihi.org) is dedicated to the task of improving the quality of the health care system. Reduction of harm and error is an important part of the IHI's mission.

The Agency for Healthcare Research and Quality (AHRQ; http://www.ahrq.gov) is the federal organization tasked with responsibility for improving the quality, safety, efficiency, and effectiveness of health care for all Americans and is an excellent resource for patient safety information.

*Journal of Patient Safety*

*The Joint Commission Journal on Quality and Patient Safety*

*American Journal of Medical Quality*

American Medical Association. Patient safety and quality tools. http://www.ama-assn.org/ama/pub/category/12582.html.

University of California at San Francisco (UCSF)-Stanford University Evidence-Based Practice Center. Making health care safer: A critical analysis of patient safety practices. http://www.ahrq.gov/clinic/ptsafety/pdf/ptsafety.pdf.

Cohen MR. *Medication Errors.* Sudbury, MA: Jones and Bartlett; 1999.

The Joint Commission. Joint commission resources: preventing medication errors: Strategies for pharmacists. http://www.jcrinc.com/ProductDetails3309.aspx.

Morath JM, Turnbull JE. *To Do No Harm: Ensuring Patient Safety in Health Care Organizations,* 1st ed. San Francisco: Jossey-Bass; 2004.

Vincent C. *Patient Safety.* Edinburgh: Elsevier Churchill Livingstone; 2006.

Wachter RM. *Understanding Patient Safety.* New York: McGraw-Hill; 2008.

# Chapter 4

# Organization Design and Management

*James T. Ziegenfuss Jr., PhD, and Thomas Biancaniello, MD, FACC*

## Executive Summary

The continuous and dedicated study of human behavior and attitudes, management systems, and organizational structures that produce high-quality medical and health care organizations is a key characteristic of successful organizations. The field of organizational design and management considers how and why people behave as they do in organized settings. The challenge for leaders in charge of quality is to design organizational structure and management systems that lead to transparent assessments of the current state of quality, continuous efforts to improve quality, and ongoing monitoring of quality of care. By providing knowledge of how and why individuals and groups behave as they do, organizational behavior theories and concepts help leaders design management systems that enable physicians and support staff to attain and maintain high medical quality.

Effective leaders are competent in the perception, motivation, and empowerment of individuals as well as group dynamics, characteristics of high-performance teams, and intergroup collaboration strategies. Effective leaders of QI also know how the diverse elements of organization design contribute to high-quality organizations. These elements include incentives and reinforcement strategies, strategic planning, development and maintenance of culture and values, and the psychological aspects of open access to information and data feedback.

In this chapter, we describe the key elements of organization design and management necessary for leaders of QI.

## Learning Objectives

Upon completion of this chapter, readers will be able to:

- describe the basics of organizational systems;
- identify the critical responsibilities of a leader in QI;
- describe the necessary steps in planning a QI program; and
- discuss the key characteristics of learning organizations.

## History

In the 1980s and 1990s, medical quality professionals and researchers led by Crosby,[1] Deming,[2] and Juran[3] examined the contributions of industrial quality improvement to see whether they could address the deficiencies of traditional quality assurance, including complexities and incompleteness of assessment without improvement.

Traditional quality assurance was historically characterized by the individual responsibility of professionals who maintained autonomy and both administrative and professional authority over quality.[4] Quality assurance teams established goals through planning, many of which were driven by responses to complaints. Failure to attain goals was indicated by retrospective performance reviews. In contrast, the TQM model for quality improvement (QI) offers a collective, management-led, team-oriented approach.[4] This model is described in detail in Chapter 1. Whole organization quality management is proactive and internally driven, a continuous seeking of the best clinical and administrative structure.

## Organizational Systems Thinking and Theories

At the start of the 21st century, theorists viewed the organization as a whole, guided by values and principles, interacting subsystems, and structures and processes of integration. An effective QI leader uses "system thinking" to coordinate these diverse systems to assess, to improve, and to control quality using organization theory and behavior principles.[5]

Ackoff defines a system as a set of two or more elements that satisfies the following three conditions: (1) The behavior of each element has an effect on the behavior of the whole. (2) The behavior of the elements and their effects on the whole are interdependent. (3) Regardless of how the subgroups of the elements are formed, each has an effect on the behavior of the whole and none has an independent effect on it.[6]

Effective clinical and administrative managers direct and lead QI, viewing organizations as *sociotechnical systems*. Pasmore explained this view by highlighting several key assumptions as noted in Table 4-1.[7]

Similarly, Kast and Rosenzweig[8] view a successful organization as open to the environment (that is, events and policy changes outside the institution are recognized and planned for) and as composed of a number of subsystems. The following descriptions are based on Kast and Rosenzweig's original work[8] and are adapted with the research and thinking of other theorists.[9] Every system is thought to be potentially comprised of five subsystems including technical, structural, psychosocial, managerial, and organizational as described below.

### 1. Product and Technical Subsystem

The product and technical subsystem includes the "core work" of health care organizations—providing medical care. The product technical subsystem varies based on the activities of the organization as a whole and of its subunits, such as departments.

TABLE 4-1   Sociotechnical View of Quality Improvement

- Quality derives from addressing whole jobs, not parts of jobs.
- Workers must have autonomy to improve quality.
- Authority for quality improvement must be delegated.
- Group rewards must support team-based quality improvement.
- Barriers to quality improvement must be eliminated.
- Quality improvement evolves by recognizing the value of people.
- Innovation for improvement supports quality.
- Quality is driven by internal and external factors.

*Adapted from:* Pasmore WA. *Designing Effective Organizations: The Sociotechnical Systems Perspective.* New York: Wiley; 1988.

For example, the technology used in hospitals differs significantly from that used in an HMO. Similarly, the products and technology of a hospital emergency room are different from those in a laboratory. The product technology subsystem is shaped by the production and delivery process, specialization of knowledge and skills required, types of equipment involved, and layout of facilities.

## 2. Structural Subsystem

This subsystem involves the ways in which the tasks of the organization are divided (differentiation) and coordinated (integration). Organization charts, position and job descriptions, and rules and procedures define the structure in a formal sense. Structure is also defined by emergent and formal patterns of authority, communication, and work flow. The organization's structure is the basis for establishing formal relationships between the clinical production process and worker psychology. For example, financial incentives are a structural tool that can be used to enhance the quality of clinical performance.[10] Many examples of flawed performance are encouraged by wrongheaded reward systems that provide structural support for undesired behaviors.[11] Informal interactions and relationships link the technical and psychosocial subsystems and can bypass the formal structure.

---

## CASE STUDY • • •

### *How Structure Enhances Function*

In 2005, Stony Brook University Hospital's risk management and quality assurance groups analyzed data from the Patient Safety Network system and closed cases and determined that the problem of *failure to rescue* needed to be addressed. Failure to rescue refers to the situation in which a patient's condition begins to deteriorate, and the response is either inadequate or too slow to reverse the clinical deterioration.

In 1995, Lee[12] and others described the formation of medical emergency teams in Australia. These teams focused on responding to patients who were clinically deteriorating to assure that they were resuscitated before they required emergent transfer to intensive care units or experienced cardiopulmonary arrest.

These medical emergency teams have become known as rapid response teams (RRTs) and are comprised of experienced clinicians who, when called to the bedside, rapidly assess the clinical situation and institute measures to reverse the status. Briefly, the elements are anyone caring for a patient is empowered to call the RRT if (1) they think the patient is deteriorating, (2) they are uncomfortable with the patient for any reason, or (3) they are uncomfortable with the response level so far. The experienced leader can be a nurse practitioner with critical care experience, senior resident or attending physician, or a respiratory therapist, because respiratory issues are common in these patients.

The quality management team and medical leadership at Stony Brook decided to pilot a RRT initially on one nursing shift on one unit. Because of the success of the initial pilot, the program was rolled out across the institution. In the first 22 months, the number of calls rose from 4 per month to 47. The number of codes for cardiopulmonary arrest fell from about 8/1000 discharges to 5.99. The Department of Anesthesia reported that their billing for out-of-operating room intubation fell by 50%. More recently, early warning systems have been implemented to advance the preventive measures to identify patients (using vital signs and other clinical assessment parameters) who require intervention by the team caring for them even before the RRT becomes necessary. Thus, risk management, quality measurement, and decision support identify the problem; quality management and medical, nursing, and hospital staff respond through the structural organization of the RRTs.

## 3. Psychosocial Subsystem

Every organization has a *psychosocial subsystem*—the psychosocial dynamics of individuals and groups that interact. Forces outside of internal structure help to establish the organization's psychological climate within which physicians, administrators, and staff perform their clinical and administrative roles and activities. As a result of this unique mix, the psychological climate differs significantly from organization to organization. Certainly, from the perspective of employees, the climate of a health maintenance organization (HMO) claims department is different, for example, from a pediatric unit or an emergency surgery. Subsystem elements may include individual behavior and motivation, status and role relationships, and group dynamics as well as the values, attitudes, expectations, and aspirations of the people in the organization. Many believe that participatory involvement of staff is central to continuous improvement.[13]

## 4. Managerial Subsystem

The *managerial subsystem* is the integrator that relates the organization to its environment; sets the goals; develops comprehensive, strategic, and operational plans; designs the structure; and establishes evaluation and control processes. Managerial activities traditionally have been described in terms of planning, organizing, developing, directing, leading, and controlling. These duties are performed through a series of management roles—interpersonal, informational, and decisional.[14] More recently, design, education, and stewardship have been viewed as core duties; thus, the managerial task includes curriculum development[15] and the training of new medical leaders.[16] Management coordinates and integrates the production, structural, psychosocial, and cultural subsystems.

## 5. Organizational Culture

*Organizational culture* is the last of the five subsystems. To be successful and to survive, organizations must meet social requirements, which comprise the goals and values of the external environment. Here we include the concept of corporate culture[17,18] and the ability to understand culture as part of clinical and administrative problem solving.[19] This subsystem links the goals and the values of the members of the organization with those of the broader society.

Each of these subsystems is a part of the architecture that must be created to stimulate quality improvement, yet each contains barriers such as inadequate clinical knowledge, poor teamwork, and resistant leadership.[20,21] They are considered internal to this perspective of the organization (i.e., hospital, private practice, HMO). There is an "external supra-system," which includes all forces outside the boundaries of the organization (defined by the five systems). These forces can include a diversity of issues, such as national and international trends, and climatic and competitive situations (some of which are barriers to quality).[22] A sample of the rich mix of these external aspects includes the following categories of environmental content:

- Economics (e.g., state and natural economy)
- Politics (e.g., cost containment, policy initiatives)
- Technology (e.g., new equipment, pharmaceuticals)
- Social and demographics (e.g., single family, aging, crime)
- Law (e.g., malpractice)
- Culture (e.g., expectations, alternative medicine)
- Natural resources (e.g., water, weather)
- Globalization (e.g., war, pollution)

These environmental factors present both opportunities for progress and can result in wasted resources if not planned for.[23]

# Responsibilities of a Leader in Quality Improvement

What, then, are the leadership requirements for quality leaders? Given that they lead their organization's quality effort, five responsibilities are essential: (1) advocacy and spokesmanship; (2) policy, planning, and vision; (3) delivery system decision support; (4) analysis and control of quality; and (5) external liaison and representation.[24] These five areas become manifested in the well-known managerial competencies of industry knowledge, vision and development skills, communication, and interpersonal ability, which are reflected in the following fundamental tasks and activities.

## Advocacy and Spokesmanship

The medical quality leader takes the lead in articulating and stimulating discussion of quality values with clinical and administrative staff. S(he) raises philosophy and purpose of quality in the institution and advocates for it in many forums, from administrative meetings to departmental specialty conferences.

## Policy, Planning, and Visioning

How well is the quality perspective represented in strategic discussions? Does it rate the prominence given to cost reduction, profit margins, and market share? Here the leader is expected to identify and to present the competitive advantages of quality and, most importantly, to lead the development of the organization's formal policies on quality management. Policy design includes consideration of objectives, quality management methods, resources, staffing, and impact. And, as an extension of this effort, the leader is responsible for creating a vision of future quality for the institution.

## Delivery System Decision Support

Most health and medical care organizations are constantly considering redesign of their delivery systems. Many are developing greater internal integration of departments and more sophisticated information systems to track patients, services, and financial transactions. Others are involved in discussions about mergers and acquisitions. Pushing integration, leaders in QI must be able to relate to many levels of authority, and bridge gaps in culture and perception.[25] The medical quality leader should play a key role in the redesign and reengineering efforts, keeping them oriented to achieve overall clinical and business quality and safety.

## Analysis and Control of Quality

Within the existing system, there is an ongoing need to identify and to collect quality data, conduct the required analyses, and act on the results to stimulate continuous improvement of the delivery system. The quality leader is expected to coordinate team processes in deciding which information is relevant and manage the subsequent data feedback.

## External Liaison and Representation

Purchasers, regulators, and consumers now seek information on institutional quality of care. We expect the chief executive to be the quality leader in a symbolic sense, establishing a culture with quality values and a continuous improvement philosophy. We expect the medical quality leader to fully represent those values in practice, helping the organization to meet and to exceed professional and accreditation standards. When industry purchasers and oversight groups request data, examples of continuous improvement gains, and detailed descriptions of quality management practice, someone must respond; the medical quality leader typically assumes the leadership and coordinating responsibility for the same.

Thus, to fulfill the responsibilities presented above, quality management leaders act in several key roles in the quality system. First, quality leaders must be *content experts*, guiding the institution to a clear and effective system based on state-of-the-art quality philosophy and methods. Second, they must act as *educators*, teaching clinical and administrative staff about the primary and advanced knowledge and skills that have developed in the quality field. The quality leader must spend time explaining why and how quality management contributes to the institution's objectives. Third, they must act as *process experts,* using interpersonal communication and group skills to lead management and clinical personnel through the development and the usage of a system of quality management. Finally, quality leaders must be able and willing to act as *evaluators,* constantly assessing the state of their quality management system and searching for ways to improve its design and operations.

The roles of the quality leader are further illustrated by using Henry Mintzberg's classic set of managerial roles.[13] Think of the quality leader as the manager of the quality process in its entirety (Table 4-2).

Successful performance in these roles requires that quality leaders have the authority and power to influence behavior (i.e., to create concerted, coordinated efforts to deliver and constantly improve quality).

## Double Track

Once we recognize that strategic decisions affect quality, it becomes clear that quality management leaders must have a voice in the *direction* of the enterprise (strategy) and in the *execution* of the strategies (operations).

The *double track* concept requires leaders in QI to attack problems and opportunities in two dimensions.[26,27] On *Track 1*, the organization level, leaders make a public and a strategic commitment to improve quality (e.g., to improve medical and health care services throughout the organization). This strategic level of the procedure requires executive leaders to promote the strategic importance of redesign and to create a vision of an improved quality future. The emphasis here is on the choice of strategy and organizational architecture (e.g., incentives, authority, relations, staffing).

*Track 2*, the project or team level track, involves very specific and operational problems (e.g., hospital discharge planning, operating room turnover, how to inform poor families about immunization and nutrition needs, placement procedures for recruiting and retaining rural physicians). Once a problem is identified, a team is formed and

TABLE 4-2   Roles and Functions in Quality Improvement

| Management Roles | Management Functions in Roles |
| --- | --- |
| ☐ **Interpersonal Roles** | |
| — Figurehead | To lead quality planning |
| — Leader | To direct and lead organization-wide quality effort |
| — Liaison | To communicate up to board, down to departments and quality teams, and outside to environment |
| ☐ **Informational Roles** | |
| — Monitor | Of quality progress |
| — Disseminator | Of quality improvement ideas and successes |
| — Spokesperson | For internal and external quality efforts |
| ☐ **Decisional Roles** | |
| — Entrepreneur | To initiate new and innovative continuous quality improvement strategies, methods |
| — Disturbance handler | To resolve quality-generated conflicts within and between teams, departments, and others |
| — Resource allocator | To distribute and develop resources for quality improvement |
| — Negotiator | To settle on quality requirements, internal and external |

*Adapted from:* Mintzberg H. *The Manager's Job: Folklore and Fact.* Boston: Harvard Business Review; 1975.

the questions quickly become the following: What is our diagnosis of the problem? What do we do? Problem-solving procedures are followed as the team crafts specific solutions. There are numerous reports of reengineering and quality improvement protocols that have been used to guide efforts, some demonstrating breakthrough success.[28]

The double track approach is based on several common purposes, including evaluation and assessment (e.g., of current service delivery, of the impact of changes); teaching and learning (e.g., about health, the effectiveness and efficiency of service delivery models); and organizational change and development (e.g., improvement in health care access). This double track approach to strategy formulation and implementation is especially successful when work is done with the vision of creating a learning organization.[29]

## High-Performing Teams

A key responsibility for leaders of quality is to enhance efficiency and effectiveness of high-performing teams, which have the following characteristics.

## Size and Structure

The team or committee size is 8 to 15. With too many participants, there literally is not enough "airtime" for individuals. Extensive minutes, subcommittees, and ad hoc groups may seem useful to address specific topics, but they can add complexity that undercuts flexibility and speed.

## Shared Vision

Co-produced by leaders and the group, the members of high-performing teams have a clear sense of where they are going (i.e., the goals of the team) and how the committee's work fits into the institution's objectives. This vision is not pre-formed but is worked out by the group.

## Focused Objectives

Specific near-term projects are clearly defined. Members have chosen objectives that are manageable within the time frame and resources available and have a defined purpose that is limited in scope. The more focused this charge, the more effective the group's output will be. Targeted and focused creativity means leaders keep to the core topic, pushing ideas that further discussion, open new options, or lead to specific actions. These are all channeled toward the group's primary mission.

## Leadership

The leader of the group attends to both the task—quality improvement—and to the relationship between team members. The leader knows that, over time, the power of the team will add significant value to the task only if attention is paid to team management. Groups require informed, participative leadership that is determined to receive input from all members. Members rapidly come to understand the style and the orientation of the leader. Leader domination, or loss of control, quickly undercuts enthusiasm and commitment.

A prepared and time-limited agenda must be distributed beforehand. Each team member must have a clear sense of what is to be accomplished at each meeting. Leaders must keep to the schedule by adhering to the predetermined meeting length while maintaining deadlines. Long meetings and missed due dates signal that the group is drifting and is likely to be ineffectual.

## Cohesion

In high-performing teams, group members are in harmony with the task and have concern for other members' values and positions. The care and nurturing of the team is the means by which the group will accomplish its agenda. Leaders manage conflict, incorporate diverse opinions, and ensure that contributions are made by all members.

They also ensure that no member dominates or pursues an agenda at the expense of the group as a whole.

## Action

Continual processing of documentation of team activities without forward movement quickly reduces member interest.

## Follow-Up

High-performing teams pay close attention to two questions: What effect did our actions have? What has been our year-long contribution to the organization's performance? Attention to outcomes of teams is both reinforcing and informative.

## Hoshin Planning

Among quality management advocates, strategic planning is often linked to the Japanese concept of hoshin planning. Although there is some effort to distinguish hoshin and strategic planning, in modern organization practice, they are quite close. The purpose of hoshin planning is to build organization performance by focusing on the quality of the medical and health care services. Hoshin is intended to link strategic planning (high-level, long-term) with operational planning and implementation (front-line, short-term) ensuring that the best visions and intentions are realized. The elements of hoshin are directed at making this two-pronged effort (strategic and operational) meld into one organization-wide, smoothly integrated endeavor.

The methods of hoshin can be captured by first noting the essential elements.

1. The QI effort is intended to be inclusive of staff at all levels. Thus, it is consistent with participative total quality management that crosses levels and functions, from top executives and managers toward all levels of personnel.

2. The leadership of the organization must buy into and visibly support the planning process, particularly the interest in listening to lower-level staff and the encouragement of cross-functional teams. The kick-off effort is the first of these high-visibility opportunities for leaders. A second opportunity is ongoing leader attention to team efforts and outcomes.

3. Resources are substantial and, as in other quality management efforts, are used to support significant training at the start, with coaching and advisory services as ongoing provision.

The planning process includes the following steps:

1. Identify key strategic issues facing the organization (e.g., patient safety).
2. Establish overall business goals and objectives (including but not exclusively quality).
3. Select strategies to address goals (e.g., quality improvement strategies).

4. Define specific objectives for each strategy.

5. Create measurement metrics and data sets for defining baselines and progress.

6. Identify key progress measures used to formally track progress.

Hoshin planning relies on a participative base that is followed by a publicizing of the progress and, as such, depends on an open culture and a lack of fear. Implementation is tracked with regular performance reviews that are charted and posted for all to see.

## Learning Organizations

How can we further understanding of overall strategy—how the patterns of quality management work as a whole? Can we do this in the organization while continuing its growth and development? Learning organizations are skilled at gaining insight from their own experiences and experiences of others and modifying the way they function based on this knowledge. They use this knowledge to continuously improve the quality of care and performance related to both strategy and operations.

In 1995, Nevis, Dibella, and Gould listed the seven key elements that illustrate the orientation of the learning system.[30] We describe these in the context QI.[29]

### Knowledge Source: Internal–External

This element emphasizes the use of knowledge derived from past internal organizational experiences by learning organizations as well as external knowledge derived from benchmarking that provides a comparative context and ideas for improvement and innovation.

### Product–Process Focus

This element emphasizes the focus on both process and outcomes to fully understand quality and to move quality forward.

### Documentation Mode: Personal–Public

This element emphasizes the dissemination of knowledge in the organization that is transparent and publicly available versus something that is available to affected individuals or groups alone.

### Dissemination Mode: Formal–Informal

This element refers to the different modes of dissemination of information and knowledge in a learning organization important to enhancing performance. These consist of both informal methods of interactions and role modeling as well as more formal methods of dissemination that may be linked to credentialing, reappointment, and performance reviews.

## Learning Focus: Incremental–Transformative

This element raises the issue of focus on incremental or corrective learning and transformative or radical learning. Enhancement of existing products or processes creates incremental or evolutionary gains versus radical gains achieved through transformation strategy such as the shift in strategic focus from acute care to prevention.

## Value–Chain Focus: Design–Deliver

This element emphasizes the focus of learning organizations on sales and service activities versus a more traditional focus on production activities.

## Skill Development Focus: Individual–Group

This element addresses focus of learning organizations on developing the team or group skills versus a traditional focus on developing individuals alone.

# Future Trends

When considering the future of the organization and management aspects of quality management, four topics come to mind:

- The growing complexity of the quality management effort coupled with the size of the investment will give rise to management challenges (e.g., who leads, how much investment in QI, pressures to adopt new technologies).

- The need to consider how leadership and management are linked to risk management, patient advocacy, safety, and other quality metrics will be increasingly raised.

- Maintaining the investment in quality management will be contested in light of continuing cost pressures and the requirement to demonstrate a return on investment.

- How improvements in quality will fit in with more general corporate organizational strategy and can be integrated into strategy formulation processes.

# References

1. Crosby PB. *Quality Is Free.* New York: McGraw-Hill; 1979.
2. Deming WE. *Out of the Crisis.* Cambridge, MA: MIT Press; 1986.
3. Juran JM. *Juran on Leadership for Quality.* New York: Free Press, 1989.
4. McLaughlin CP, Kaluzny AD. Total quality management in health: Making it work. *Health Care Manage Rev.* 1990;15(3):7–14.
5. Flood AB, Fennell ML. Through the lenses of organizational sociology: The role of organizational theory and research in conceptualizing and examining our health care system. *J Health Soc Behav.* 1995;extra issue:154–169.

6.  Ackoff RL. *Creating the Corporate Future.* New York: Wiley; 1981.

7.  Pasmore WA. *Designing Effective Organizations: The Sociotechnical Systems Perspective.* New York: Wiley; 1988.

8.  Kast FE, Rosenzweig JE. *Organization and Management: A Systems and Contingency Approach*, 4th ed. New York: McGraw-Hill; 1985.

9.  Ziegenfuss JT. *Organization and Management Problem Solving: A Systems and Consulting Approach.* Thousand Oaks, CA: Sage Books; 2002.

10. Goldfarb S. The utility of decision support, clinical guidelines, and financial incentives as tools to achieve improved clinical performance. *Jt Comm J Qual Improv.* 1999;25(3):137–144.

11. Kerr S. On the folly of rewarding A, while hoping for B: More on the folly. *Acad Manage Exec.* 1995;9(1)7–16.

12. Lee A, Bishop G, Hillman KM, Daffurn K. The medical emergency team. *Anesth Intens Care.* 1995;23:183–186.

13. Hammermeister KE. Participatory continuous improvement. *Ann Thorac Surg.* 1994;58(6): 1815–1821.

14. Mintzberg H. The manager's job: Folklore and fact. *Harv Bus Rev.* 1975;49–61.

15. Colenda CC, Wadland W, Hayes O, et al. Training tomorrow's clinicians today—managed care essentials: A process for curriculum development. *Am J Manag Care.* 2000;6(5):561–572.

16. Blair JD, Payne GT. The paradox prescription: Leading the medical group of the future. *Health Care Manage Rev.* 2000;25(1):45–58.

17. Smircich L. Concepts of culture and organizational analysis. *Adm Sci Q.* 1983;28:339–358.

18. Schein EH. *Organizational Culture and Leadership.* San Francisco, CA: Jossey-Bass, 1985.

19. Lundberg CC. Knowing and surfacing organizational culture: A consultant's guide. In: Golembiewski RT, ed. *Handbook of Organizational Consultation.* New York: Marcel Dekker; 1993.

20. Ziegenfuss JT Jr. Organizational barriers to quality improvement in medical and health care organizations. *Qual Assur Util Rev.* 1991;6(4):115–122.

21. Langlais RJ. Recognizing organizational impediments to the total quality management process. *Best Pract Benchmarking Healthc.* 1996;1(1):16–20.

22. Reinertsen JL. Collaborating outside the box: When employers and providers take on environmental barriers to guideline implementation. *Jt Comm J Qual Improv.* 1995;21(11):612–618.

23. Reinhardt UE. The United States: Breakthroughs and waste. *J Health Polit Policy Law.* 1992;17(4):637–666.

24. Ziegenfuss JT. Five responsibilities of medical quality leaders. *Am J Med Qual.* 1997;12(4):175–176.

25. Ashkenas RN, Fracis SC. Integration managers: Special leaders for special times. *Harv Bus Rev.* 2000;78(6):108–116.

26. Ziegenfuss JT. *The Organizational Path to Health Care Quality.* Ann Arbor, MI: Health Administration Press; 1993.

27. Ziegenfuss JT. Toward a general procedure for quality improvement: The double track process. *Am J Med Qual.* 1994;9(2):90–97.

28. Nackel JG. Breakthrough delivery systems: Applying business process innovation. *J Soc Health Syst.* 1995;5(1):11–21.

29. Shortell SM, Jones RH, Rademaker AW, et al. Assessing the impact of total quality management and organizational culture on multiple outcomes of care for coronary artery bypass graft surgery patients. *Med Care.* 2000;38(2):207–217.

30. Nevis EC, Dibella AJ, Gould JM. Understanding organizations as learning systems. *Sloan Manage Rev.* 1995;36(2):73–85.

## Additional Resources–Further Reading

Anctil B, Winters M. Linking customer judgments with process measures to improve access to ambulatory care. *Jt Comm J Qual Improv.* 1996;22(5):345–357.

Begun, JW, Luke RD. Factors underlying organizational change in local health care markets, 1982–1995. *Health Care Manage Rev.* 2001;26(2):62–72.

Blumenthal D, Edward N. A tale of two systems: The changing academic health center. *Health Aff.* 2000;19(3):86–101.

Bossidy L. The job no CEO should delegate. *Harv Bus Rev.* 2001;79(3):46–49, 163.

Checkland P. *Systems Thinking, Systems Practice.* New York: Wiley; 1981.

Chisholm R, Ziengefuss JT. Applying the sociotechnical systems approach to health care organizations. *J Appl Behav Sci.* 1986;22(3):315–327.

Goldsmith J. The Internet and managed care: A new wave of innovation. *Health Aff.* 2000;19(6): 42–56.

Hofer TP, Hayward RA, Greenfield S, et al. The unreliability of individual physician "report cards" for assessing the costs and quality of care of a chronic disease. *JAMA.* 1999;281(22):2098–2105.

Kazandjian VA, Thomson RG, Law WR, Waldron K. Do performance indicators make a difference? *Jt Comm J Qual Improv.* 1996;22(7):482–491.

Keating CB. A systems-based methodology for structural analysis of health care operations. *J Manag Med.* 2000;14(3–4):170–198.

Kritchevsky SB, Simmons BP. Continuous quality improvement: Concepts and applications for physician care. *JAMA.* 1991;266(13):1817–1823.

Landon BE, Wilson IB, Cleary PD. A conceptual model of the effects of health care organizations on the quality of medical care. *JAMA.* 1998;279(17):1377–1382.

Lesser CS, Ginsburg PB. Update on the nation's health care system, 1997–1999. *Health Aff.* 2000;19(6)206–216.

Maxwell C, Ziegenfuss JT, Chisholm RF. Beyond quality improvement teams: Sociotechnical systems theory and self-directed work teams. *Qual Manage Health Care.* 1993;1(2):59–67.

McLaughlin CP. Balancing collaboration and competition: The Kingsport, Tennessee experience. *Jt Comm J Qual Improv.* 1995;21(11):646–655.

Nackel JG. Breakthrough delivery systems: Applying business process innovation. *J Soc Health Syst.* 1995;5(1):11–21.

Prahalad CK, Krishnam MS. The new meaning of quality in the information age. *Harv Bus Rev.* 1999;77(5):109–118, 184.

Schein EH. Culture: The missing concept in organizational studies. *Admin Sci Q.* 1996;11(2): 229–240.

Schein EH. Three cultures of management: The key to organization. *Sloan Manage Rev.* 1996;38(1): 9–20.

Schein EH. *Organizational Culture and Leadership,* 3rd ed. San Francisco: Jossey-Bass; 2004.

Shortell SM, Bazzoli GJ, Dubbs NL, Kralovec P. Classifying health networks and systems: Managerial and policy implications. *Health Care Manage Rev.* 2000;25(4):9–17.

Weil TP. Management of integrated delivery systems in the next decade. *Health Care Manage Rev.* 2000;25(3):9–23.

Wyszewianski L. Quality of care: Past achievements and future challenges. *Inquiry.* Spring 1988;25(1):13–24.

Chapter 5

# Medical Informatics

*Louis H. Diamond, MB, ChB, FACP, and Stephen T. Lawless,*
*MD, MBA*

## Executive Summary

Health care delivery is largely dependent on an information exchange between the patient and the health care professional, and among health care professionals. The field of medical informatics examines the structure, the acquisition, and the use of health care information. The components of an information infrastructure include the medical record, including elements such as a personal health record and continuity of care records; point-of-care decision support tools; and performance measurement systems. All these components support individual patient management and the management of patient populations.

Technology can enhance health care quality and quality measurement in various ways. It increases accuracy and timeliness, enables up-to-date evidence and decision support systems to be used at the point of patient care, improves coordination of information among clinicians and between patients and clinicians, and enhances the capacity to collect and report information on performance.[1] Furthermore, technology can determine the extent to which health plans can capture relevant data for quality measures and the degree to which policy makers are able to measure improvement in health care over time.

Access to patient health records and electronic medical literature about best practices and population-based data can promote the practice of evidence-based medicine. In addition, electronic "alert systems" can aid decision making. Finally, technology offers the capacity to increase the speed with which new information about clinical practices is generated and disseminated to practitioners, especially regarding the provisions of performance information, a necessary but insufficient requirement to facilitate provider behavioral change and system re-engineering.

This chapter provides an overview of medical informatics necessary for an executive in charge of quality management.

*Learning Objectives*

Upon completion of this chapter, the reader should be able to:

• describe the national initiatives driving the development of a national health care information infrastructure;

• describe the components of a national health care information infrastructure;

• identify the basics of the U.S. coding classification systems;

• discuss the electronic medical record (EMR) and its impact on safety and quality; and

• describe the principles and components of decision support systems.

## History: The Evolution of Medical Informatics in the United States

The prevailing opinion is that the use of information technology (IT) in health care is lagging 10 to 15 years behind IT in other industries such as banking, manufacturing, and airlines.[2] Health care providers, faced with an unprecedented era of competition and managed care, are actively exploring opportunities to use IT to improve the quality, the safety, and the cost of health care. In recent years, annual spending on health care IT has been estimated at $12 billion to $14 billion.

The recent history of medical informatics in the United States is shown in Table 5-1. In the IOM report *Crossing the Quality Chasm* there was a clear imperative to develop the health information infrastructure in the United States to support quality and safety. They felt that in the absence of a national commitment to build a national health information infrastructure, the progress on quality improvement will be painfully slow.[3] In 2004, David Brailer was appointed to lead the Office of the National Coordinator for Healthcare Information Technology (ONCHIT), a new office created within the Department of Health and Human Services. Created by executive order of President Bush, ONCHIT's primary task was to create the U.S. National Health Information Network (NHIN) with time lines for achieving certain goals. The framework articulated four overarching goals: inform clinical practice, interconnect clinicians, personalize care, and improve population health. Specific strategies have been developed for each of these goals.

The American Health Information Community (AHIC) has been established under the aegis of ONCHIT. AHIC has a broad-based charge directed at engaging public and private sector stakeholders to provide for strategic direction and to facilitate implementation of the building of a national health information infrastructure.

Further exponential growth in medical informatics is expected as the health care industry implements electronic medical records (EMRs), upgrades hospital information systems, sets up intranets for sharing information among key stakeholders, and uses

| TABLE 5-1 | Recent History of Medical Informatics in the United States |
|---|---|
| **Key Date** | **Element–Milestone** |
| May 3, 2001 | First e-health federal legislation introduced. |
| Oct 2001 | Consolidated Health Informatics Initiative launched. |
| Nov 2001 | Debut of the National Health Information Infrastructure. |
| June 2002 | E-prescribing federal legislation introduced. |
| Nov 2002 | IOM reports released. |
| Dec 2003 | Medicare Prescription Drug, Improvement, and Modernization Act of 2003 (Public Law 108-173) passed—contains demonstration projects. |
| Jan 2004 | Health Information Technology (HIT) highlighted in President Bush's State of the Union address. |
| April 2004 | President Bush unveils executive order on HIT. |
| May 2004 | Office of the National Coordinator for Healthcare Information Technology (ONCHIT) established. |
| June 2004 | President's Information Technology Advisory Committee releases a report titled *Revolutionizing Healthcare through Information Technology*. |
| July 2004 | HHS launches the HIT decade, a strategic framework for a national health information infrastructure. |
| May 2005 | HHS releases final report of the HIT Leadership Panel. |
| June 2005 | HHS releases Request for Proposals to cover standards setting, the NHIN, a certification commission, and privacy and security. |
| Oct 2005 | HHS releases proposed rules on e-prescribing. |
| Aug 2006 | AHIC announces the formation of multiple work groups. |
| Aug 2006 | HHS releases the final e-prescribing regulation. |
| Oct 2006 | HIT Standards Panel (HITSP) recommends the first round of interoperability specification. |

public networks such as the Internet for distributing health-related information and for providing remote diagnostics. Along with these drastic changes and the new approach to health care, the point-of-care applicability of health–medical informatics has experienced significant growth in the last few years.[2]

# Essential Components of a Health Information Infrastructure

## Data Sources

Patient-specific data is needed to provide patient care services, to support a robust point-of-care decision support system, and to support quality performance metrics. Identifying the measure specification then mapping to the data elements and HIT standards required to collect and store the data provides a road map for action. Both AHIC and expert panels at the NQF have started that process, as of mid-2007.

Data are potentially available from a wide variety of sources: claims data; hard copy information, such as medical records; and formal systems that provide payment information, such as claims and survey data. Some of these data are available to organizations electronically through internal systems.

## Data Definitions

The quality of data in an information infrastructure depends on the degree to which the data captures—with completeness, detail, and accuracy—the concepts of interest. In health care information systems, a *data set* refers to a commonly agreed upon collection of data elements that are used for defining a clinical domain. Terms associated with this process include *terminology*, *classification*, and *nomenclature* and are largely used interchangeably. Terminology refers to health care terms and their definitions that are communicated numerically through combinations of coded data elements. Technically, the more precise nomenclatures are aggregated to form classifications, and the continuum from one to the other is referred to collectively as terminology.[4]

Presently, over 150 clinically related classification systems, nomenclatures, dictionaries, terminologies, vocabulary lists, and code sets are used in the United States.[4] Each classification system was designed to meet a specific need (e.g., physician reimbursement). Each system differs in the extent to which it is general, disease specific, or domain specific. Furthermore, the content and the structure of the classification systems vary. Building the future information infrastructure will require developing a system of measures that are universally standardized and understood.[5,6] Standard terminology enables data capture to proceed in a structured manner, facilitating the collection of information and enhancing the ability to perform data analyses.

## Coding Classification Systems

It is essential to adopt classification systems and standards for the data elements, including data transmission, storage, and analysis, and use of the data. The following is an outline of some of these classifications.

### International Classification of Diseases (ICD)

The health care system in the United States uses the International Classification of Diseases, Version 9, and Clinical Modification for Use in the United States (ICD-9-CM) as its official system of assigning codes to diagnoses and procedures related to hospital use. The classification system is used for provider reimbursement, quality review, and benchmarking measurements. Based on the World Health Organization's (WHO) classification system, the 10th revision of the International Classification of Diseases (ICD-10) is used to code and classify mortality data from death certificates. In the United States, the

National Center of Health Statistics (NCHS) and CMS manage the system and modify it to meet the particular needs of the nation's evolving health care system.[7] Current efforts are under way to complete a clinical modification of the ICD-10 diagnoses (ICD-10-CM). Additionally, CMS has already completed the development of an ICD-10 companion procedural classification system (ICD-10-PCS). This classification system has the adaptability and flexibility to accommodate new technologies more quickly than has been the case with ICD-9-CM procedural classification updates.

## Current Procedural Terminology (CPT)

A system used for classifying clinical procedures and services performed by physicians is the Current Procedural Terminology, fourth edition (CPT-4).[8] The system is developed under the auspices of the American Medical Association (AMA) and is used by accreditation organizations; by payers for administrative, financial, and analytical purposes; and by researchers for outcomes studies, public health initiatives, and health services research. Efforts are under way to develop the next generation of CPT (CPT-5). The new system is designed to respond to the challenges of the Health Insurance Portability and Accountability Act of 1996 (HIPAA) and supports electronic interfaces. Specifically, CPT-5 is designed to communicate easily with demographic information systems, electronic health records, and analytical databases of varying levels of detail. It is anticipated that CPT-5 will be the standard for reporting physician's services under HIPAA regulations.

## Systematized Nomenclature of Medicine (SNOMED)

Used in more than 40 countries, the Systematized Nomenclature of Medicine (SNOMED) represents a broad array of health care concepts.[4] SNOMED was created for indexing the entire medical record, including signs and symptoms, diagnoses, and procedures. It is being adopted worldwide as the standard for indexing medical records information. SNOMED may be used for disease management, health services research, outcomes research, and quality improvement analyses. It is promoted as a system through which detailed clinical information can be shared across specialties, sites of care, and various information system platforms.

## Unified Medical Language System (UMLS)

Developed by the National Library of Medicine, the UMLS provides an electronic link between clinical vocabularies and medical literature from disparate sources.[4] The goal is to develop a means whereby a wide variety of application programs can overcome retrieval problems caused by differences in terminology and the scattering of relevant information across many databases. For example, UMLS eases the linkage between computer-based patient records, bibliographic databases, factual databases, and expert systems. The National Library of Medicine distributes annual editions, free of charge under a license agreement, and encourages feedback, which promotes expansion of the database. The UMLS Semantic Network contains information about the types or categories to which all

Metathesaurus concepts have been assigned (e.g., disease or syndrome, virus) and the permissible relationships among these types (e.g., virus causes disease or syndrome).[4]

### Health Level Seven (HL7)

HL7 is a not-for-profit standards development organization, accredited by the American National Standards Institute (ANSI), whose mission is to provide standards for the exchange, the management, and the integration of medical data that support clinical patient care and the management, the delivery, and the evaluation of health care services.[9] HL7 supports an application protocol for the electronic exchange of clinical and associated administrative data. The application communicates orders, referrals, diagnostic results, and visit notes across health care entities. HL7 may be thought of as a standard for the data structure for records that are sent between individual systems, the content and terminologies of which are constantly being revised and expanded to meet various health informatics needs.

### Logical Observation Identifiers, Names, and Codes (LOINC)

The development of a system known as Logical Observation Identifiers, Names, and Codes (LOINC) originally focused on a public use set of codes and names for electronic reporting of laboratory test results.[10] It has been expanded to encompass a database of names, synonyms, and codes, and it can also capture clinical measurements, such as EKG data. LOINC content is continually expanding to include more direct patient measurements and clinical observations. LOINC data are available from the Regenstrief HL7 Website.[10] An extensive review of these needed standards is described in a recent IOM report entitled *"Patient Safety: Achieving a New Standard of Care."*[11]

### Diagnosis-Related Groups (DRGs)

In DRGs, patients are categorized into one of 498 groups by diagnosis, major surgical procedure, age, sex, and presence of a complication or comorbidity. Diagnosis-related groups, which are homogeneous groupings with respect to hospital charges and length of stay, are best known for their use in Medicare hospital payments, but they are also used for comparative hospital cost and efficiency studies.

### All Patient Refined Diagnosis-Related Groups (APR-DRGs)

This methodology uses the DRG case-mix schema with diagnosis-based severity levels to account for a patient's level of illness. Although the underlying DRG structure is resource-based, clinical judgment and empirical testing are used in designing and validating the severity levels.

## Data Transmission

Data transmission is a critical component of the information infrastructure. Issues surrounding secure data transmission include a transmission mechanism; format and content standards; a unique identifier to ensure that records are appropriately assigned to the correct individual; assurance of data confidentiality; and mechanisms to ensure data security. These issues have received widespread attention, as epitomized in the 1996 HIPAA legislation, which is described in detail in Chapter 9.

Data that are stored in different formats need to be mapped and translated. In the absence of standardization, translations often must be performed manually, which is costly and raises the potential for error. The standardization of data formats and elements can eliminate this cumbersome step. At present, many health care organizations rely on HL7 for this standardization function.

A controversial and important issue in health care data transmission is the use of a unique patient identifier. The unique identifier can enable an individual's lifetime experience with the health care system to be accessed electronically. The development of a unique health care identifier was included in the 1996 HIPAA legislation to maximize the potential of electronic health care data systems. However, several years ago Congress placed the national patient identifier on hold due to implementation complexities.[12] There are substantial privacy concerns surrounding the use of a unique patient identifier. For example, using social security numbers could inadvertently cause a linkage to personal information data unrelated to health care. A variety of non-numeric approaches to a unique identifier, including DNA prints and thumbprints, have been proposed[12]; however, it appears that even the transmission of this information would require translation to a numeric base. These and other privacy concerns have caused the issue of a unique patient identifier to be placed on hold indefinitely.

## Health Information Exchange (HIE)

*HIE* is the exchange of health information, and in the use of the term, implies the exchange is occurring electronically. The components of HIE include communication with clinicians—for example, with physicians by hospitals and laboratories or between clinicians and their patients. Basic requirements for HIE include the existence of HIT standards and data definitions that are standardized across settings and clinicians, so as to facilitate data collection and transmission. Regional health information organizations and other entities will require organization and a governance structure to facilitate HIE and will need to define a business model to initiate and sustain functions and activities. The kind of activities sponsored by an HIE include secure communication; sharing of patient results; e-consultation; patient summary information, including a medication record and, eventually, a full-fledged personal health record; and formulary and related decision support for both the health care professional and the patient.

## Data Storage

Storage methods have important implications for their use. The storage method should allow providers, patients, managers, and others to access the data in a format that meets their particular needs. The separate functions of three common data storage systems—operational data stores, data warehouses, and data marts—must be recognized.

The operational data store offers real-time data, is process-oriented, provides data in textual output, and serves a distinctly operational function. Operational data stores drive *clinical decision support systems* (CDSS), which are clinical consultation systems that use population statistics combined with expert knowledge to offer real-time information to clinicians. The focus of these systems is individual patient management, and patient-specific information is included in the analysis. Such systems are useful in day-to-day operational decisions.

Data warehouses differ fundamentally from operational data stores in that data warehouses are designed for strategic decision support rather than for operational decision support.[13-16] The data warehouse maintains historical data summarized in analytical aggregates, and its analytical paths are loosely structured to facilitate varied investigations. The data warehouse offers graphical presentations of information and serves a managerial function.

A data warehouse is a centralized repository of a single copy of corporate integrated data that comes from a variety of sources; serves the needs of the entire organization; and typically includes data from sources such as claims, providers, pharmacies, laboratories, and materials management. The data warehouse has analytic and querying functions and can specifically analyze clinical and financial information for purposes of utilization review, component cost evaluation, and clinician performance evaluation.

Often referred to as "health care archaeology," data warehouses generally store information from a 3- to 5-year period and are used to evaluate clinical and financial performance in groups of patients after care has been given. Although the data warehouse holds important information for population analysis, the large volume of data that it contains often makes it cumbersome. The data warehouse has a primary purpose of storing and constructing data marts to support specific purposes.

Data marts are department oriented, smaller in scope, less expensive to manage, and less time consuming to construct. They are built for a specific analytical purpose and serve a small group of analysts. A data mart offers improved accessibility to the data and few maintenance issues for the database administrator. Once data have been aggregated in a data mart, they are easier to manipulate for analysis.

## Data Analysis

The ability to collect and maintain health care information and its exchange over an information infrastructure is essential for analytic support of quality measurement and management. Further details on quality measurement and reporting measures are described in Chapter 2. Today, many well-known and respected methodologies can be integrated in a data warehouse for use in outcomes studies, provider profiling analyses, payment development, and forecasting. Among the better known risk-adjustment methodologies are DRGs, APR-DRGs, disease staging, episodes, episodic treatment groups, episode groupers, resource use methods, ambulatory clinical conditions, and diagnostic cost groups. These risk-adjustment and severity-of-illness methods have been designed to quantify risk for hospitalized patients. They are used to calculate hospital payment and to monitor clinical efficiency and hospital costs.

## Disease Staging

Disease staging consists of two risk-adjustment methodologies. The first is predicated on the progression of disease and involves documenting increasing levels of severity, known as *disease stages*. More than 600 diseases are distinguished, and patients may fall into more than one disease category based on the number of diagnoses recorded on a hospital claim. The disease staging charge, length of stay, and mortality scales form the basis of the second risk-adjustment technique. The scales are patient-level forecasts of expected resource use and in-hospital mortality.

### Episodes

The unit of analysis for episode risk-adjustment techniques is a clinically defined course of illness. Inpatient and outpatient claims and encounters are associated with an episode. An episode ends after a period during which no claims are encountered, and the patient is assumed to have recovered from an acute illness or condition. Chronic episodes typically are open-ended and accumulate claims for the duration of the study period.

### Episodic Treatment Groups (ETGs)

The methodology of ETGs uses homogeneous treatment episodes that categorize patients by disease condition and medical or surgical intervention. Cost weights profile the efficiency of treatment of patients by physicians.

### MEDSTAT Episode Grouper (MEG)

In the MEG methodology, episodes are constructed around the disease or medical condition of a patient, regardless of treatment. Each episode is constructed from disease staging by disease categories and severity. The method enables users to compare and contrast the timing and appropriateness of medical interventions.

### Resource Use Methods

Diagnosis-based risk-adjustment methods calculate risk-adjusted payments to physicians and hospitals. These resource-use methods are employed in disease management and provider profiling studies.

### Ambulatory Clinical Groupings (ACGs)

The methodology of ambulatory clinical groupings (ACGs) is constructed by using the diagnoses and patient demographics found on inpatient and outpatient claims. Patients are categorized into a single ACG based on demographic information and their diagnoses over the study period. In a few cases, an ACG is related to specific medical conditions; however, most of the groups are broad (e.g., chronic medical, unstable).

*Diagnostic Cost Groups (DCGs)*

The original purpose of the diagnostic cost group (DCG) risk-adjustment methodology was to design a method for administering prospective ambulatory care payments to physicians. Initially, diagnoses from inpatient and outpatient claims are categorized into 543 diagnostic groups. These groups are further collapsed into 118 hierarchical condition categories (HCCs). Based on a patient's HCC, statistical forecasts reflect the incremental cost of each condition. Populations may be stratified by demographic attributes (age, sex, insurance status, and various socioeconomic attributes), as well as by measures of health status. This case-mix adjustment methodology predicts a population's past or future health care utilization and costs. Various grouping applications, such as ACGs, DCGs, and disease staging applications may be used. These types of categorizations and analyses are important for quality improvement investigations because they level the playing field by taking into account the intensity of illness of the patient under care.

Various types of adjustment approaches are in common use. ACGs use claims and encounter information to group individuals who are likely to have similar resource requirements, on the theory that level of health is associated with level of health care resource use. ACGs use ICD-9 diagnosis codes and demographic information to assign individuals to one of 83 mutually exclusive categories that are found to have similar resource requirements. Similarly, DCGs require ICD-9 diagnosis data from claims and encounter data, where groupings are based on expenditures of samples of Medicare recipients. Disease staging is a way of adjusting for variation in patient clinical severity, which is based on the concept that diseases naturally progress through stages. The assumption is that these stages can be measured independently of the services provided.

# Electronic Medical Record (EMR)

The effect of the aging baby boomer population on the economy and the health care system has been exhaustively reported. The changes driven by demographics will be the result of a variety of forces, including issues related to technology that will shape health care over the coming years. The EMR is a means to establish a virtual data–information center to serve as a dynamic repository to enhance the ability of the advisory bodies and the staff to collect and to analyze data. This virtual data–information center can serve as a vehicle to promote and to disseminate standardized data definitions and best practices to providers, consumers, and others interested in quality improvement efforts nationally and internationally.

Currently, over 60% of consumers believe patients will receive better care and errors will be reduced if information is shared among doctors and researchers via electronic systems. Over 50% of consumers believe health care costs could also be reduced. Over 90% of consumers think that patients should have some access to their own EMRs maintained by their physician; 67% believe that the benefits of an EMR outweigh the privacy concerns. However, only about 25% of these consumers report that their physician uses some form of EMR.[17]

The positive expectation but lack of experience with an EMR exposes a general knowledge gap for most patients and health care providers. Some of the ideal specifications of an EMR are listed in Table 5-2.

An EMR allows the substitution of classical human dependent steps. System and human errors are the principal barriers to determining which practices are best. Significant variances from desired outcomes often result from such errors. Reducing these variances from desired outcomes will come about only if an infrastructure is established to facilitate data collection and analysis and to put the results of those analyses to use.

Monitors, smart pumps, bar coding, and other new technologies are aspects of care now moved to the bedside but not yet consistently integrated within the EMR. This lack of integration of the bedside technologies and the EMR places an additional burden on health care workers and may create distractions that impede their performance of their clinical roles and responsibilities.

## Computerized Physician Order Entry (CPOE)

*CPOE* (see Chapter 3) is a process of electronic entry of physician instructions for the treatment of patients. These orders are communicated to the appropriate departments, the support staff, and other providers over a computer network to decrease delay in order completion and to eliminate errors of legibility. Experience indicates that medication errors are reduced when CPOE is utilized.[18-22] Depending upon the level of application sophistication, additional benefits could occur in terms of medication prescription and safety and prevention of order duplication.

Most hospitals in the United States have an application designed for nonphysicians to enter orders electronically from the physician's written orders in the patient chart, but a minority utilizes CPOE. Quality studies with the use of nondecision support CPOE have shown that while legibility errors are eliminated, significant numbers of errors with prescription writing are not related to legibility (Figure 5-1). Physicians

---

**TABLE 5-2   Global Expectations of an EMR**

Provides an electronic documentation of all patient events, both episodic and recurrent.

Serves as a single source of all information for the patient, trended from conception to death.

Allows data availability on a just-in-time basis for all care providers who are directly working with the patient.

Allows data views that accommodate the needs of unique users without creating data pollution.

If combined with a data warehouse, the data from multiple EMRs and applications can be aggregated in order to provide a means to determine best practice, appropriate guidelines for care, and population health improvements.

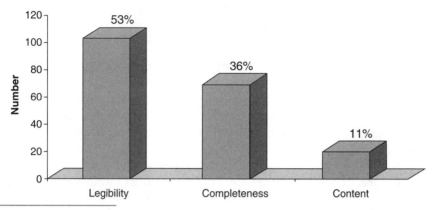

**Figure 5-1** Errors Related to Hand-Written Prescriptions and Potentially Prevented by CPOE

*Source:* This figure is provided courtesy of Nemours and originated from a quality review of written prescriptions over a one-month period in 2001. http://www.nemours.org.

have been slow to adapt to CPOE because it increases the time required to write an order; it may force definitively directed decision making depending upon the granularity of the order structure; and it requires a nonmedical skill (typing) that some older practitioners do not have. Recent evidence[23,24] demonstrates that the EMR can help to significantly reduce medical errors, especially those associated with writing paper prescriptions.

## Decision Support Systems

Decision support systems are another class of computer-based information systems that ideally are evidence-based, integrated with the EMR, and include knowledge to support decision-making activities.[18,20] Decision support can take the form of "reminder cues" or may suggest or require that an action be performed. The degree of force behind a reminder is a function of the message desired. A "soft stop" reminder still allows variation of care, while a "hard stop" will require an action or inaction and may even require a specific choice from a series of predetermined selections. The downside to reminders–alerts is the phenomena of "alert fatigue" and decreased response to an alert. Clearly, some balance is required as to decision support tools, because without them preventable errors are occurring.

Diagnostic decision support is beneficial. In several ways, an allergy alert when ordering helps reduce adverse drug reactions. More sophisticated decision support tools embedded within the EMR require significant and expensive customized coding. Published studies report the value of decision support[25,26] through the use of reminders and forced data entry.

# EMR's Impact on Quality and Safety

A fully integrated EMR can serve as a cohesive force in that alignment that creates a health care system. The EMR can serve as the organized portal by which patients and their families can receive more than just episodic care, including the following, as outlined by the Foundation for Accountability[27]:

- The basics: understanding the health care delivery system in general and how to access services.

- Staying healthy: obtaining recommended preventive health care services and learning positive health behaviors.

- Getting better: meeting needs in acute care settings.

- Living with illness: coordinating effective care for patients with chronic and complex conditions in ways that link the quality of care.

- Changing needs and end-of-life care: addressing the physical, psychological, social, and spiritual needs of patients and families regarding the long term of life with disability, and the impact of the death of a child in a society where it is perceived as an extraordinary and unnatural event.

The EMR is enhancing practice efficiency as reflected by the significant improvement in the availability of patient records and the information contained in that record. This availability facilitates the patient receiving health information and laboratory results in a timely fashion, while allowing the physician to make accurate decisions regarding medical advice and medication management. As is being demonstrated nationally, the amount of "transactional friction" (those steps or processes that do not improve the financial bottom line, the error-free rate, or number of process steps) within the health care system has been estimated to account for more than 30% of total health care expenditures.[23]

Errors are prevalent in health care; medication errors are reported to occur in the range of 55% of patients, with another 12% potentially experiencing an adverse drug event as a direct result of a medication order error.[18] Several types of IT will likely reduce the frequency of medication errors. CPOE and decision support tools can substantially decrease the frequency of serious errors.

The work flow requirements of individual units must be analyzed before technologies like CPOE can be properly developed and implemented.[19] The implementation of EMRs, CPOEs, and decision support tools is not risk-free. Studies highlight that CPOE technology is still evolving and requires ongoing assessment of "systems integration" and "human–machine interface" effects—both predictable and unpredictable—on patient care and clinical outcomes.[28]

Others have reported positive results on patient processes and clinical outcomes. Patients treated with both the initial and the modified CPOE system were similar for all measured characteristics. With the modified CPOE system, there were significant reductions in orders for vasoactive infusions, sedative infusions, and ventilator management.

The EMR is considered a strong tool that improves documented communication. Can the EMR also be utilized to improve aspects of care (e.g., handoffs)? Recent reports[29] show that significant errors that would have impacted patient care, in fact, resulted from sign-out transfer data elements (weight, medications, allergies) not directly integrated from an EMR. Introduction of an EMR-based sign-out sheet designed by the same residents eliminated the errors.[30] EMR-based clinicians[31] were significantly more likely to address a variety of routine health care maintenance topics including diet, identification of psychosocial issues, smoking, lead risk assessment, exposure to domestic or community violence, guns in the home, behavioral or social developmental milestones, infant sleep position, breastfeeding, poison control, and child safety. Interestingly, many EMR users reported reduced eye-to-eye contact with patients and increased duration of visits. All users recommended continued use of the system. Use of the EMR in this study was associated with improved quality of care.

EMR adoption is clearly in its infancy, but its use and the concomitant experience are growing. Adaptation to the EMR has been slightly hindered by cost considerations and functionality that may not be inherent to each user. This is balanced by the clear reduction in medical errors (especially medication errors) as a result of the EMR and CPOE decision support. Further progression of the EMR as a tool to help integrate care is still in development.

Advanced decision support, along with integrated records that link visit information within an EMR, can also be utilized to improve care coordination. Triggered prompts to guide decision support will allow just-in-time identification of disease progression, allow reassessment of care, facilitate patient-centered involvement, and obtain information regarding real and perceived impact on outcomes and quality of life in the short and the long term.

---

## CASE STUDY • • •

### *Facilitation of Care Coordination via a Well-Functioning EMR: A Fictitious Case of Recognition, Treatment, and Follow-Up of Childhood Obesity Using an EMR*

A patient is seen for an annual physical examination. During the examination, a height and weight are recorded in the EMR. Once entered, a risk-adjusted body mass index (BMI) is automatically calculated along with a percentile rating. For this patient, a BMI that is above the 95th percentile is highlighted. The elevated BMI result is linked to the blood pressure recording. If the blood pressure is also at a certain threshold (i.e., 90th percentile), an alert is triggered for the provider that allows identification of obesity and hypertension. The provider is then reminded to add key data elements into the history and physical examination record. Laboratory testing to screen for active disease progression is ordered and transmitted as a request to the appropriate laboratory (i.e., fasting glucose and lipid profile) in order to screen for diabetes mellitus and cardiovascular heart disease. A follow-up visit is arranged within the

EMR, synchronized with the return of the laboratory results. A medical action plan that is individualized for each patient is documented and includes educational materials for the patient to understand, community resources to help with management, activity advice, and dietary advice. These resources are obtained both via tools embedded within the EMR and linked to Internet Websites that allow easy access. Follow-up blood pressure, patient weight, and physical activity logs can be uploaded in the EMR, either by direct patient home access to the EMR or by direct interfaced digital results from home equipment (i.e., scales, blood pressure, glucometer). Patient diaries prompted at both fixed and variable intervals for outcomes and quality-of-life indicators are also entered into the EMR via the Internet in such a fashion that the provider can match treatment goals to progression. These results can be viewed and treatment plans reassessed as needed, not solely at the time of the next appointment but also based upon decision support algorithms that track marginal goal progression and alert automatically when either compliance and/or goals are at risk.

## Personal Health Record

The *personal health record* (PHR) is a component of one of the three articulated goals of the national HIT agenda. It is an e-record of an individual's health information. The patient is the primary user and manages and shares the information. Other dimensions of the PHR are to make the information available to members of the health care delivery team and to facilitate information sharing, thus avoiding errors and miscommunication and otherwise providing for the opportunity to improve patient outcomes.

From a structural perspective, PHRs fall into three categories: (1) stand-alone, with information entered by the patient; (2) integrated with, directly connected to, and populated by an EMR and electronic hospital record (EHR); and (3) payer or employer populated, with claims and other data. The latter two categories can be interchangeable and should have a feature that allows for the patient to add information (e.g., medications taken, quality-of-life metrics, blood pressure levels taken at home). Regardless of the mechanism used to collect it, PHR data should be organized and displayed in a user-friendly manner, with information that is useful to and useable by the patient and members of the health delivery team.

Some of the barriers to adoption of a PHR are patient concerns about privacy and security; provider concerns about the accuracy of the data (and concomitant liability); lack of integration of the data into EMRs and work flow; lack of HIT standards and interpretability; and lack of awareness on the part of consumers and health professionals. Additionally, there are issues of creating a sustainable business model to cover the costs of maintaining a PHR.

## Evaluating an Information Infrastructure

The evaluation of an information system should focus on technical efficiency and the ability to meet the needs of the end user. To achieve technical efficiency, the components of the information infrastructure should be evaluated to determine what is expected and to explore how well the infrastructure is performing. To satisfy the end user, the evaluation should center on whether the needs and the perceptions of consumers, physicians, organizations, and governments are being met.

On the technical side, the following types of questions need to be asked:

- Have key data sources been accessed?
- Are standards in place for data content, structure, and coding?
- Is information sufficiently detailed to answer critical questions?
- Are data transmitted among organizations with relative ease, and do the systems interact well?
- Are data stored in the most appropriate ways to facilitate extraction and analysis?
- Are the systems user-friendly?
- Are reports generated with ease and speed?
- Are the data current and accurate?
- Is the Internet interface user-friendly?
- Are the data secure? Are multiple firewalls used? How difficult is it for an unauthorized person to access the data?

For the end user, answers to the following questions are important:

- Is the investment cost-effective?
- Is the system efficient?
- Are the data sources adequate to answer key questions?
- To what extent does the system contribute to the ability to measure and to promote quality?
- Is the investment leading to increases in user satisfaction?
- Are outcomes improved?
- What is the return on investment?
- Is practice variation reduced?
- Are the information and communication needs of patients, physicians, and managers being met?

## Barriers to Development of an Adequate Health Information Infrastructure

Although an electronic information infrastructure holds much promise for improving the quality of health care services, the rapid development of IT faces many technical, financial, and political barriers. Technical barriers include the complexity, decentralization, and fragmentation of the health care system and the lack of standards for terminology, coding, and data transmission. Financial obstacles include the relative absence of payment incentives tied to quality measurement, the inability to demonstrate a convincing return on investment for large IT undertakings, the low capital investment in IT, and the fear among health care organizations of exchanging information with competing providers. A variety of political barriers also exist, such as industry regulation issues, intellectual property issues, and concerns about confidentiality and privacy.

The highly complex and fragmented nature of the U.S. health care system hampers the ability to collect and analyze data within and across organizations. Data collection and analysis processes entail combining data from various sources and making comparisons using different information systems and processes. Measuring the quality of care requires access to a wide range of information from varying sources; however, health care programs, plans, and providers may use different software packages for different requirements (e.g., claims processing, utilization management, and provider credentialing), and basic data, such as patient identifiers, may vary between health plans and sometimes even between different providers within a plan. Moreover, many providers are not part of large health care systems with high-powered information networks. The U.S. health care system is highly decentralized. There is little consistency in standards for terminology, data coding, or data transmission across providers or vendors. Although some standards developed by organizations accredited by the ANSI are in fairly wide use, much variation exists, because many organizations modify these standards for their own purposes. Moreover, vendors for each clinical system often have unique classification systems. The absence of uniform data standards is a significant barrier to using technology to improve quality, because it impedes the aggregation of data from local to national levels. Measuring and interpreting outcomes, providing continuous quality improvement, and allocating limited resources to optimize quality and effectiveness requires comparable data.[32]

Currently, a main obstacle to IT development in health care is the low expenditure on these systems compared with that in other industries. For example, the expenditure on IT is $543 per employee in the health sector, whereas it is $12,666 per employee among securities brokers. Health care ranks 38th out of 58 industries in its investment in IT.[3]

One reason for this low expenditure may be the difficulty in proving the return on investment. Another reason may be that investments in large data warehouses have failed to meet expectations.[13,14] Investment in quality improvement technology may be limited in part because payment incentives do not encourage it.[2] Fear of sharing information with competitors may also slow progress toward development of an integrated information infrastructure because providers may believe that they are jeopardizing their competitive position. Further, providers may not want to change their data management systems to accommodate more standardized ones because they believe that the cost of doing so is unnecessary.

In the political arena, data privacy and confidentiality issues are highly visible. Regulation is another important policy issue and potential roadblock. The Food and Drug Administration has been debating whether to regulate clinical decision software as a medical device. Other concerns relate to intellectual property (copyright and patent) issues and liability.[32]

## Health Information Technology and Return on Investment

There is growing recognition that HIT provides benefits such as reduced error and adverse events rates, improved quality and efficiency, and the ability to coordinate care and conduct needed biosurveillance. For each of these dimensions, the literature still remains mixed, making it difficult to generalize positive findings from examples of benefit conducted in academic centers, utilizing homegrown, incrementally built HIT systems.

There is sparse literature documenting the capital costs and the costs of implementation and maintenance of a health information network. Kaushal et al. have concluded the capital costs to be $156 billion, with $48 billion in annual operating costs.[33] Chaudhry et al. have emphasized the lack of generalizability and related issues in their systematic review of the impact of HIT on quality, efficiency, and costs.[34] A study by Hillestad et al. claimed that more than $81 billion could be saved annually by adopting EMR systems and networking.[24]

These dollar figures, computed at a national level, are not easily extrapolated to a regional and local level. Additionally, the costs are unevenly borne by different stakeholders, and the benefits are spread across various stakeholders, often unrelated to those that bear the expenditures. The role of the public and the private sectors regarding these financial matters is still in a state of evolution.

## Future Trends

We believe that medical informatics will play a key role in the future of quality improvement and patient safety. The proliferation of new technology and information systems will reduce or eliminate many serious threats to patient safety and will become more cost-effective, ensuring more widespread use of information systems in small group practices and hospitals. These systems will also help health care providers become more productive and create a fulfilling work environment that promotes job satisfaction, recruitment, and retention. As pay-for-performance programs go into effect, the health information infrastructure will need to be developed to provide accurate quality measurements. Next-generation decision support systems will enhance point-of-care services and ensure provision of evidence-based care.

Although we did not discuss other branches of medical informatics (e.g., telemedicine, imaging systems, patient informatics, remote monitoring, and robotics) in this chapter, these areas are critical to enhancing patient-centered care and safety, and, we believe, these areas will proliferate in the next few decades.

# References

1. Chassin MR. Is health care ready for six sigma quality? *Milbank Q.* 1998;76(4):565–591, 610.
2. Chassin MR, Gavin RW, National Roundtable on Health Care Quality. The urgent need to improve health care quality. *JAMA.* 1998;280(11):1000–1005.
3. Institute of Medicine. *Crossing the Quality Chasm: A New Health System for the 21st Century.* Washington, DC: National Academies Press; 2001.
4. National Library of Medicine. Unified Medical Language System (UMLS). http://www.nlm.nih.gov/research/umls. Accessed October 8, 2008.
5. Bakken S. An informatics infrastructure is essential for evidence-based practice. *J Am Med Inform Assoc.* 2001;8(3):199–201.
6. McDonald CJ. Need for standards in health information. *Health Aff.* 1998;17(6):44–46.
7. Centers for Disease Control and Prevention (CDC), National Center for Health Statistics. Classification of Diseases and Functioning and Disability. http://www.cdc.gov/nchs/icd9.htm. Accessed October 1, 2008.
8. American Medical Association. CPT (Current Procedural Terminology). http://www.ama-assn.org/ama/pub/category/3113.html. Accessed October 9, 2008.
9. HL7. What Is HL7? http://www.hl7.org. Accessed October 9, 2008.
10. The Regenstrief Institute. Logical Observation Identifiers, Names, and Codes. http://www.regenstrief.org/loinc. Accessed October 1, 2008.
11. Institute of Medicine, Committee on Data Standards for Patient Safety. In Aspden P, Corrigan JM, Wolcott J, Erickson SM, eds. *Patient Safety: Achieving a New Standard for Care.* Washington, DC: National Academies Press; 2004.
12. Unique Patient Identifiers. Future Initiatives Having HIPAA Implications. http://www.medscape.com/viewarticle/506843_5. Accessed October 9, 2008.
13. Bush D. Why is data warehousing failing us? *Managed Healthcare News.* 2000;16:6.
14. Breen C, Rodrigues LM. Implementing a data warehouse at Inglis Innovative Services. *JHIM.* 2001;15(2)87–97.
15. Inmon B. Data mart does not equal data warehouse. November 1999. http://www.dmreview.com/dmdirect/19991120/1675-1.html. Accessed October 9, 2008.
16. Ramick DC. Data warehousing in disease management programs. *JHIM.* 2001;15(2):99–105.
17. Bright B. Benefits of electronic health records seen as outweighing privacy risks. *Wall Street Journal Online/Harris Interactive Health-Care Poll*, November 29, 2007. http://online.wsj.com/public/article/SB119565244262500549.html.
18. Kaushal R, Bates DW, Landrigan C, et al. Medication errors and adverse drug events in pediatric inpatients. *JAMA.* 2001;285(16):2114–2120.
19. Ali NA, Mekhjian HS, Kuehn PL, et al. Specificity of computerized physician order entry has a significant effect on the efficiency of workflow for critically ill patients. *Crit Care Med.* 2005;33(1):110–114.
20. Kaushal R, Barker KN, Bates DW. How can information technology improve patient safety and reduce medication errors in children's health care? *Arch Pediatr Adolesc Med.* 2001;155(9):1002–1007.
21. Leape LL, Bates DW, Cullen DJ, et al. Systems analysis of adverse drug events. *JAMA.* 1995;274(1):35–43.
22. Kripalani S, LeFevre F, Phillips CO, et al. Deficits in communication and information transfer between hospital-based and primary care physicians: Implications for patient safety and continuity of care. *JAMA.* 2007;297(8):831–841.

23. Walker J, Pan E, Johnson D, et al. The value of health care information exchange and interoperability. *Health Aff.* January 19, 2005. http://content.healthaffairs.org/cgi/content/full/hlthaff.w5.10/DC1. Accessed October 10, 2008.

24. Hillestad R, Bigelow J, Bower A, et al. Can electronic medical record systems transform healthcare? Potential health benefits, savings and costs. *Health Aff.* 2005;24(5):1103–1117.

25. Balas EA, Weingarten S, Garb CT, et al. Improving preventative care by prompting physicians. *Arch Intern Med.* 2000;160(3):301–308.

26. Morris AH. Treatment algorithms and protocolized care. *Curr Opin Crit Care.* 2003; 9(3):236–240.

27. Foundation for Accountability. Patient-Centered Care Measures for the National Health Care Quality Report, 2001. http://www.markle.org/resources/facct/doclibFiles/documentFile_168.pdf. Accessed March 25, 2005.

28. Han YY, Carcillo JA, Venkataraman ST, et al. Unexpected increased mortality after implementation of a commercially sold computerized physician order entry system. *Pediatrics.* 2005; 116;1506–1512.

29. Frank G, Lawler LA, Jackson AA, et al. Resident miscommunication: Accuracy of the resident sign-out sheet. *J Healthc Qual.* 2005;27(2):4–14.

30. Frank G, Lawless ST, Steinberg TH. Improving physician communication through an automated, integrated sign-out system. *JHIM.* 2005;19(4):68–74.

31. Adams WG, Mann AM, Bauchner H. Use of an electronic medical record improves the quality of urban pediatric primary care. *Pediatrics.* 2003;111(3):626–632.

32. Moran D. Health information policy: On preparing for the next war. *Health Aff.* 1998; 17(6):9–22.

33. Kaushal R, Blumenthal D, Poon EG, et al. The costs of a national health information network. *Ann Intern Med.* 2005;143(3):165–173.

34. Chaudhry B, Wang J, Wu S, et al. Systematic review: Impact of health information technology on quality, efficiency, and costs of medical care. *Ann Intern Med.* 2006;144(10):742–752.

## Additional Resources–Further Reading

Health Information Privacy and Security Collaborative (HISPO): http://www.hss.gov/healthit
American Health Information Community (AHIC): http://www.hhs.gov/healthit/community/background
Agency for Healthcare Research and Quality (AHRQ): http://www.AHRQ.gov
Health Resources and Service Administration (HRSA): http://www.hrsa.gov
National Institute of Standards and Technology (NIST): http://www.nist.gov
Health Information Technology Standards Panel (HITSP): http://www.hitsp.com
National Quality Forum. *CEO Survival Guides Series. Personal Health Records.* 2007 ed. http://www.nqfstore.org/store/category.aspx?categoryID=10.

### HIT Standards (Abbreviated)

LOINC, Laboratory testing coding: http://www.loinc.org
SNOMED CT3, Clinical text coding (within EMR): http://www.cap.org
UMLS, Overall Coded Medical Language: http://www.nlm.gov
ICD-10, Diagnosis/Procedure Coding (hospitals): http://www.who.int/en
CCR, Continuity of Care Record (for snapshot of patient for next caregiver): http://www.astm.org

CDA, Clinical Document Architecture (for discharge summaries and progress noted): http://www.h17.org

HIPAA, Transaction Sets (837, 857). http://www.cms.hhs.gov/TransactionCodeSetsStands/02_TransactionsandCodeSetsRegulations.asp

NCPDP, Pharmacy: http://www.ncpdp.org

DICOM, Radiology images: http://www.nema.org

CDISC, Exchange of clinical trial information: http://www.cdisc.org

HL7, Messaging standards for clinical–administrative data communication across medical devices–systems: http://www.h17.org

# Chapter 6

# Economics and Finance in Medical Quality Management

*Donald Fetterolf, MD, MBA, FACP, and Rahul K. Shah, MD, FAAP*

## Executive Summary

Professionals engaged in quality improvement (QI) are frequently asked to evaluate issues involving medical errors, patient satisfaction, utility and efficacy of emerging technologies, and to make a variety of other critical decisions related to the adequacy and appropriateness of care.[1-3] These issues are inextricably entwined in the economic fabric of our society. The greatest current challenge is to balance a business-oriented focus on short-term financial outcomes with a medically oriented focus on the long-term gains created by QI methods.

It is widely held that "higher quality costs less," and quality improvement efforts have been proposed as one method for reducing skyrocketing health care costs. As quality managers are asked to select medical management activities that are cost-effective, it is becoming apparent that higher quality sometimes costs *more*—although perhaps less than the same thing done poorly. As the next generation of quality management evolves, medical quality managers, along with other institutional leaders, must confront a trade-off between some elements of quality and the costs that can be borne by a society that continuously seeks to improve the health of its population.[4-7] Indeed, newer approaches for reviewing the value of quality initiatives are multidisciplinary and consider financial, clinical, operational, and a variety of intangible variables.

Finally, increasing pressure is being applied by the payer community to document the return on investment (ROI) of quality improvement activities. Large-company benefit managers typically demand to know what the ROI is for clinical quality improvement activities and whether or not these activities are worth purchasing.[8] The lesson for physicians who are responsible for quality regarding the economics, the finance, and the politics of health care is that a major planned, or even unexpected, change in any one of these fields will likely affect the other two. Predicting the result of these dynamics becomes infinitely more complicated when the outcome is not definitive—or even tangible—but rather is a consequence of shifting resources that affect the cost of health care, alter the quality of health care, or impinge on access to health care. Even then, the dynamics can be viewed from, or measured at, multiple levels that are not necessarily consistent or even comparable.[9]

111

This chapter reviews the fundamentals of the economics, finance, and politics of medical quality in national, state, and local terms and illustrates how these three fields interact.

## Learning Objectives

Upon completion of this chapter, readers should be able to:

- discuss the general business principles and key concepts in economic theory that the medical quality practitioner must understand;

- understand the key financial and accounting concepts and detail how these tools are used in new models of care delivery analysis and operations;

- discuss the economic and the policy events that caused the government to become involved with medical quality; and

- outline the roles of American values and health policy in which medical quality practitioners should approach their tasks.

## Historical Perspective

The evolution of medical quality efforts in the United States has in many ways paralleled similar developments in the business world. Quality-oriented activities have progressed from an inspection-based approach to more modern, data-driven, analytic methods and principles of statistical quality control. At the same time, the approach of medical quality professionals has become increasingly entwined in a variety of business activities. The evolution of this process can be divided into the stages of quality assurance, statistical quality control and CQI, and outcomes-focused analysis, all of which are addressed in detail in Chapters 1, 2, and 7.

Physician-level public reporting of clinical outcomes has been discussed for a number of years, but with increasing shifts to consumer-driven health care programs and better availability of data, the public is questioning why more information is not made accessible. Subtle, important nuances in interpreting health care data that are well known to statisticians and physicians are viewed skeptically by eager but less sophisticated advocates of public reporting as roadblocks in the public's quest to find good physicians and to eliminate ineffective or dangerous practitioners. That public pressure will accelerate public disclosure is certain, with uncertain results. Simultaneously, consolidating large data sets in enterprise data warehouses in government and insurer organizations has led to the possibility that informatics-driven evaluation of process may build on the previous activities as well. Predictive modeling, data mining, and the application of a variety of sophisticated techniques for locating and abstracting information related to medical quality initiatives are being utilized at unprecedented rates.

# Basic Concepts in Business and Economics

Providing an in-depth knowledge of business economics and finance is beyond the purview of a single chapter in a book directed at fundamental training for quality professionals. Yet, this knowledge has become increasingly important for all health care professionals. The main categories of economics, accounting, and finance will be reviewed briefly, particularly as they relate to quality professionals.

## Economics

A common misunderstanding among clinically trained health care professionals is that economics is all about money. In fact, economics focuses on the creation, the evolution, and the delivery of *value*, which may include nonmonetary elements such as labor forces, factors that alter the business cycle, the influence of history, and the general thoughts and motives of the population in the aggregate.

Business schools divide the study of economics into *macroeconomics* and *microeconomics*. Macroeconomics typically deals with the "big picture" in the structure and the performance of the industrial market and the behavior of society at large. The money supply and how it affects wages, prices, employment, inflation, and long-term growth and productivity make up a major part of this topic. Macroeconomics focuses primarily on the behavior of the economy as a whole and its total output and activity at the national or international level. It also deals with these activities over time and studies how they affect the wealth of nations and overall business cycles.

Macroeconomics usually focuses on overall markets rather than on a specific small region or product, but it can be applied locally. Students of the subject recognize that it is an inexact science that has developed a variety of approaches. Keynesian economics was developed in the earlier part of the 20th century, and its tenets were frequently quoted as guiding principles until the late 20th century. The Keynesian approach has since been supplemented by a variety of theoretical constructs that continue to evolve.[10]

Regulation of the monetary supply by the Federal Reserve Board presents a "monetarist" approach to economics that is relatively recent and that has been fueled by complex econometric computer models. Considerable disagreement arises among various schools of economics as to what the best approach may be, how the market responds to various drivers, and what a government's best course of action may be. These theories are also influenced in part by the political views of individual analysts, who might emphasize the role of business and organizations over the perceived need to improve the quality of life for the general public, for example.

The health care system as a whole is clearly an issue in macroeconomics, now that the overall cost of health care is 16% to 17% of the gross domestic product of the United States. As the health care delivery system has expanded, it has assumed an increasingly large role in the overall economy, including manufacturing, labor, and the economies of governments. Economists have noted a close relationship in practice between consumption spending and disposable income.[11] Clearly, current trends in the use of disposable income in health care spending are unsustainable from a mathematical perspective. Historical changes in the U.S. economy during economic recessions have resulted in considerable pressure on large businesses to reduce health care expenditures as they become an increasing portion of a company's expenses, and in a way that makes the company less competitive in world markets. One of the most salient examples of such problems driving down the financial competitiveness of a multinational corporation is the problem faced by General Motors, one of the "big 3" automakers in the United States, whose responsibility for health benefits for current and retired workers is over $50 billion! An understanding of the structure of macroeconomics is useful for quality professionals as the economic environment in health care becomes increasingly complicated.

The second portion of the course work in economics focuses on microeconomics, or "the economics of the firm." In contrast to macroeconomics, which centers on industrial market structure and performance, microeconomics focuses on the effects of these various forces on individual firms and regions or market segments. In health care, microeconomic studies focus on individual physician practices, the workings of hospital markets and service areas, and the nuances of physician payment systems. Market demand and demand curves are of interest to various kinds of individual companies seeking to set the price and the volume of services they offer. This area of economics is clearly relevant to a medical care system that has been growing during the past 5 decades, particularly with the support of government subsidies.

Microeconomics is also concerned with the behavior of individuals as they relate to an organization. How individuals view the price of a company's service is related to the utility that they attribute to these services. In organizations that appear to offer commodities—and health care is increasingly being positioned as a commodity—payers at the individual or business level may be indifferent to which provider is used and will move to higher prices or different providers only when more complex relationships alter demand, such as changes in co-pay structure or high-deductible health plan designs.

Microeconomic analysis can evaluate consumer behavior in the purchase of health care services. Large insurance carriers conduct market research and then mathematically review ways in which consumer behavior can be altered, such as through various types of charges and perceived quality. For example, insurers and payers are interested in the types of incentives that may change the likelihood that consumers will seek health services, particularly as this likelihood relates to pricing—the so-called price elasticity of demand (Table 6-1).

The response of individuals in *monopoly* or *monopsony* markets is also of interest to large insurance carriers, in both *highly concentrated* and *unconcentrated* labor markets. In a monopoly, a seller of services represents a dominant or unique vendor of services. Prices for services can be set higher than in more competitive markets. In highly concentrated markets, which have only a few insurers for a region, individuals and businesses may complain that this effect is what makes their premiums high. They may state that high

TABLE 6-1   Price Elasticity of Demand Among Purchasers of Health Insurance Services

Insurers—indeed sellers of many products—note that certain price points will move customers in the direction of their product. For example, insurers and managed care organizations report that as little as a $10 per member per month (PMPM) out-of-pocket cost can cause a consumer to shift from one type of health provider to another. Physicians often are firmly convinced that their patients will come to them forever because they believe that the definitive bond is the relationship between the doctor and the patient. Actual practice, however, suggests that a consumer will shift to a different physician to obtain a savings of $8 to $10 PMPM. The easier it is for the patient to shift plans and networks, the more "elastic" the relationship is between individuals and the choice of purchasing services by a given physician. Many factors affect the elasticity of demand. Examples are (1) the presence of equivalent substitutes (the perception among some patients that all doctors are equal or offer commodity services); (2) the penetration of the product into the community (patients will pick HMOs if many are available in the marketplace but may be less inclined to do so when managed care develops in an indemnity market) or perceived differences in quality; and (3) the income profile of the consumer purchasing the product.

"barriers to entry" in the market prevent the competition from lowering prices. Similar complaints arise when a "sole community provider" of health care services, such as a regional rural hospital, negotiates higher fees for its services with a health plan.

In a monopsony, the purchaser of services represents a unique or dominant position in the market. The federal government with respect to Medicare services can be thought of as a monopsony, as it might be a dominant employer in a region. The effects in this case also concern the public and the government officials as the costs of health care rise. This issue is of concern to physicians, who represent a segment of the labor force that must contract with various organizations. For example, the behavior of primary care and specialist physicians likely varies in different types of markets, depending on the level of the physician's market control. In markets with a dominant insurer and an oversupply or undersupply of a particular type of physician specialty, these factors greatly affect the physicians' interpretations of how aggressive they can be with the payer. Physicians who are in short supply and in high demand can negotiate higher-than-normal fees for their services. Physicians who are in more plentiful supply might feel more downward pressure on their fees; they become "price takers." In markets that are highly fragmented across many payers, the behavior of physicians and insurers would vary according to whether physician specialties are over- or underrepresented.

Clearly, the leverage that a payer or a health plan has over physicians is also related to economic forces. How closely physicians are tied to a health plan directly influences their need or their desire to participate in mandated quality initiatives. The economics of the behaviors of patients and providers has been studied with much interest. Textbooks that combine micro- and macroeconomics and a solid knowledge of the health care system are worth reviewing by medical care professionals of all types—and by quality professionals in particular.[6,7,12-15]

In conclusion, the importance of economics to health care professionals in general, and to quality managers in particular, is becoming increasingly evident as the overall effect of the health care system on the general economy becomes more prominent and more acute. Understanding economic forces and their relationship to the business community is an important capability, if not compulsory skill, needed at all levels of management in health care organizations. Training in economics can be obtained through graduate-level courses, although several less difficult avenues are possible. Intensive short courses offered by graduate business schools, brief introductory training sessions offered through professional societies, and instructional audiotapes are available.[17] Health economics has developed into a specialty in its own right, and entire texts are available on the subject.[12,17,18]

## Accounting

Why do quality management professionals need to develop a working knowledge of accounting, let alone take a course in this subject? The reason is that basic accounting principles are used in a variety of analyses and are the "language of business." Accounting is the main method used to record business transactions and to present them to other business professionals to communicate cost and movement of money. Although health professionals need not perform accounting procedures, they still must understand and appreciate basic accounting principles in much the same way that those pursuing internal medicine rather than surgery must have a thorough knowledge of anatomy.

### Types of Financial Reporting Tools
Medical quality managers are called on to review and to understand the significance of a wide variety of financial information. Financial information can take many forms in a health plan or hospital.[19]

**Financial Statements** *Financial statements* include the balance sheet, the income statement, the statement of cash flow, and similar documents. These are used to communicate with external entities, such as the Internal Revenue Service, auditors, investors, banks, and state governments.

Important features of financial statements are often expressed as ratios. These ratios include the *current ratio* (current assets divided by current liabilities), the *quick ratio* (current assets minus inventories divided by current liabilities), and various forms of debt and profit ratios. These statistics provide an estimate of how "solid" the company is or whether its assets are sufficient to cover the debt it carries. Similar ratios reflect the return on activity of the company; for example, ROI, *return on assets* (ROA) or *return on equity* (ROE), and *earnings per share* (EPS) of stock are typically used. In these statistics, the amount of net earnings or revenue is divided by the numbers used for summarizing the asset base, outstanding equity, or by outstanding shares of stock, respectively. For medical managers, the most frequently requested statistic is the ROI—the amount of money returning to the organization for the financial investment in an initiative. This statistic is particularly difficult to obtain accurately in medical management activities in which clinical returns often are not easily converted to financial equivalents.

**Balance Sheets**   A *balance sheet* presents a financial picture of a company or organization at a fixed point in time (Table 6-2). As such, it is a "snapshot" that records the organization's assets, liabilities, and, in the case of a publicly owned company, the owner's equity.

TABLE 6-2   Sample Balance Sheet

| Balance Sheet: ABC Medical Corporation | |
|---|---|
| **Balance Sheet** | **As of December 31** |
| **Assets** | |
| *Current Assets* | |
| Cash | $50,000 |
| Accounts Receivable | 35,000 |
| Total Current Assets | $85,000 |
| *Noncurrent Assets* | |
| Land | $200,000 |
| Medical Office Building | 1,579,000 |
| Equipment (net of accumulated depreciation) | 250,000 |
| Total Noncurrent Assets | $2,029,000 |
| **Total Assets** | **$2,114,000** |
| **Liabilities** | |
| *Current Liabilities* | |
| Accounts Payable to Suppliers | $25,000 |
| Salaries Payable to Employees | 32,000 |
| Taxes Owed | 52,000 |
| Total Current Liabilities | $109,000 |
| *Noncurrent Liabilities* | |
| Notes Payable to Lenders | $150,000 |
| **Total Liabilities** | **$259,000** |
| **Shareholders' Equity** | |
| Common Stock | $1,500,000 |
| Retained Earnings | 355,000 |
| **Total Shareholders' Equity** | **$1,855,000** |
| **Total Liabilities and Shareholders' Equity** | **$2,114,000** |

In its simplest form, the balance sheet provides a picture of how big the company is and how much of its size is owed to others. It typically presents several derivative statistics, often depicted as ratios (e.g., current ratio, quick ratio), that show how much and to what degree a company's assets and liabilities are committed to hard assets, outstanding loans, liabilities of other types, taxes, and other areas. The liquidity of the organization's assets, or the ability of the company to move cash, is an important part of this statement.

**Income Statements**    Probably more important to practicing managers than the financial statement or the balance sheet is the *income statement*, which is useful in the ongoing evaluation of a business or modeled initiative. In the standard income statement, sources of revenue are listed at the top of the sheet, expenses are listed below in numerated "line item" form, and a final net income is given at the bottom. This format is typically used to communicate the sales efforts of the organization or the company and the costs that must be subtracted from profits.

Quality professionals should also recognize that while recording information in accounting ledgers they must consider the *accounting basis*. Many physicians or nurses initially entering hospital or managed care environments are accustomed to the cash accounting, or *cash-basis accounting*, used in their practices. Here, revenue and costs are recognized in the month or period in which they occur. For a variety of reasons, large operating concerns, for which revenue and expenses may not match neatly in each month, follow *accrual-based accounting*. In this approach, companies record revenue and expenses in the period in which they were incurred, regardless of the time in which money may have actually changed hands or in which a check was received. Accrual-based accounting requires regular upkeep of accounting ledgers but is more appropriate than cash-based accounting for organizations that have cash flows that are not closely temporally linked.

In health care, real profitability and future growth are assessed with *earnings before interest and taxes (EBIT)*. This element is important in the income statements of both for-profit and not-for-profit health care companies because it identifies the "real" earnings of a company. The expanded concept of *earnings before interest, taxes, depreciation, and amortization (EBITDA)* is often used in income statements when estimates of cash profitability are desired. Interest, taxes, depreciation, and amortization are used in financial and tax accounting to reduce taxable profits. Thus, EBIT and EBITDA represent earnings that are available for reinvestment in the company and are important in estimating profitability, the capital structure of the company, and other important concepts in both taxed and tax-exempt organizations.

**Statements of Cash Flows**    Another important accounting reporting tool is the *statement of cash flows* (Table 6-3). This statement typically shows the sources of cash received by the organization or the company and provides an overview of whether the organization can shift its liquid assets around in its operations. This statement is typically of more interest to financial managers than to medical quality professionals, but its existence and general structure are worth reviewing.

TABLE 6-3   Sample Statement of Cash Flows

| Cash Flows: ABC Medical Corporation | |
| --- | --- |
| Statement of Cash Flows | For Current Year |
| **Operations** | |
| Cash Flow from Operations | $1,662,000 |
| **Investing** | |
| Sale of Noncurrent Assets | $0 |
| Acquisition of Noncurrent Assets | –30,000 |
| Total Cash Flow from Investing | $–30,000 |
| **Financing** | |
| Issue of Partner Stock | $50,000 |
| Dividends | –2000 |
| Total Cash Flow from Financing | $48,000 |
| **Net Change in Cash Flow** | $1,680,000 |

The statement of cash flows accounts for the cash moving through the organization from *operating, investing,* and *financing activities.* Selling goods or services is the predominant method for realizing operating cash flows. The acquisition of noncurrent assets, particularly property and equipment, makes up the investing section of the statement and is needed for the company to function. Finally, the company's efforts to obtain cash for short- and long-term use are described in the financing section of the statement.

Statements of cash flows assess the effect of ongoing operations on the liquidity of the corporation and describe the relationships among the various components. The statement may reveal that the company is out of balance with respect to cash inflows and outflows, a situation that can precipitate a "cash crisis," in which insufficient cash is available to meet the needs of the corporation. Alternatively, the statement may show the availability of too much cash, which suggests that the company is not making the best use of this resource.

**Annual Reports**   A company's *annual report* is designed to provide an overview of the company and the company's financial position and is directed from the president to persons involved in running the company, to stockholders, and to stakeholders. The report typically contains annual and quarterly financial statements, including a balance sheet, an income statement, and a statement of cash flow, along with other information, such as a letter from the company president and a statement from an independent auditor. People who review these documents are often most interested in the supplementary information at the end of the report, particularly the management letter provided by the independent auditor. Areas of concern documented in the management letter may raise "red flags" among those concerned about the organization's assets and its future prospects for growth and performance.

## Types of Accounting Systems

**Generally Accepted Accounting Principles**  Many of the accepted accounting principles in the United States have been developed through a centralized method called *generally accepted accounting principles* (GAAP). Annual reports, balance sheets, and similar types of accounting documents are prepared using GAAP. These principles are set by general approval from three main formal organizations: the American Institute of Certified Public Accountants (AICPA), the Securities and Exchange Commission (SEC), and the Financial Accounting Standards Board (FASB). These organizations gained influence in the development of accounting principles during the mid-to-late 20th century. These accounting principles, however, have not been adopted universally, and in many countries, other, sometimes completely different, accounting systems may be operating. Recently, several international organizations have sought to standardize financial accounting methods for use in international commerce.

**Statutory Accounting Standards**  Accounting and financial reporting can also include a variety of *statutory accounting standards* that are developed by government agencies. Similar to more standard financial accounting principles used by accountants and the managerial accounting principles used in companies, statutory accounting principles are standardized, often on a national or state-by-state basis, and are used by departments of health and departments of insurance to regulate health plans. Like income tax forms, these statutory forms contain a variety of financial and sometimes clinical or utilization information that is useful to the state or the federal government. Statutory information may be calculated using certain algorithms that better allow state regulators to determine effectiveness, solvency, and similar aspects of a health plan or hospital management.

The efforts of the National Association of Insurance Commissioners (NAIC) to develop "model acts" that outline standardized recommendations for writing legislative and statutory requirements have contributed significantly to generating order in the health care industry. Widespread adoption of these principles has helped foster a relatively consistent approach across the country in the insurance industry.

**Managerial Accounting**  In addition to offering financial accounting, business schools typically offer a course in *managerial accounting* that focuses more on the day-to-day operations of the corporation. The approaches used in managerial accounting are often not part of GAAP but are adopted regularly by organizations for internal use. The purpose of these approaches is to provide senior management with a clear view of financial events in the company.

An important concept in managerial accounting is *contribution income,* which is reflected in the *contribution income statement.* In this variation of the income statement, revenues and expenses are listed on a per-unit-of-production basis. Thus, the revenues from an individual item (such as a surgical procedure or service) are linked with its expenses to show the *contribution margin,* or profit, from the sale of each item. Fixed expenses or fixed overhead must also be taken into consideration, and these items are presented later in the contribution income statement. The value of this approach is that the overall profit can be calculated easily once the "break-even point" is known (i.e., the point at which the contribution margin from the sale of a certain number of widgets equals the amount of the fixed expenses or overhead). The application of this approach to medical management initiatives is clear. If a certain medical cost saving per member per month (PMPM) is anticipated from an intervention that costs a known amount, the number of individuals who need to be treated per month to cover the monthly cost—or the overall cost and overall fixed expenses of the initiative (the break-even point)—can be calculated. From these figures, the amount of profit from each additional member treated per month (the *marginal profit)* can be calculated. *Marginal cost* is calculated in a like manner (Table 6-4).

Other organizations outside of the government statutory accounting efforts also set out to develop standard accounting processes. Many of these represent managerial accounting approaches to evaluate specific problems in the industry in which they are found. A recent example of such an effort includes the DMAA: The Care Continuum Alliance's initiative (DMAA Outcomes Guides, DMAA Disease Management Program Evaluation Guide) to standardize the reporting for estimating the economic impact of

TABLE 6-4   Study Discussion and Example: Differences Between a Regular Income Statement and a Contribution Income Statement

Standard income statements generally reflect sources of revenue and expenses and then define the difference as net profit.

### Form of a Regular Income Statement

| | |
|---|---|
| **Revenues** | |
| Revenues | $100 |
| | |
| **Expenses** | |
| Variable Expenses | $60 |
| Fixed Expenses | $20 |
| **Profit (Loss)** | $20 |

A contribution income statement presents variable revenues and expenses separately from fixed expenses and notes the relationship between the volume of business activity and the ultimate profitability of the organization.

*(continues)*

**TABLE 6-4**  *continued*

### Form of a Contribution Income Statement

|  | PMPY | Total |
|---|---|---|
| Members Affected |  | $50,000 |
| **Revenues** |  |  |
| Variable Revenues/Savings | $7 | $350,000 |
| **Expenses** |  |  |
| Variable Expenses/Unit | −$5 | −$250,000 |
| **Contribution Margin** | $2 | $100,000 |
| **Fixed Expenses** |  | $46,000 |
| **Profit (Loss)** |  | $54,000 |

In this example, the break-even point would occur when 23,000 members were treated; at this point, the revenues would equal the remaining expenses (that is, 23,000 members times the contribution margin of $2 per member would generate $46,000, the amount needed to meet the fixed expenses). Above this point, the marginal profit of the effort would accrue at a rate of $2 per member per year.

PMPY = per member per year.

disease management programs. These are particularly relevant to quality managers because disease management evaluation is often included within the realm of accreditation programs. Another example of standardized reporting of what are essentially financially related statistics include the Healthcare Effectiveness Data and Information Set (HEDIS) utilization and financial reporting data elements.

A second important concept in managerial accounting is the relatively recent method called *activity-based cost accounting* (Table 6-5). In this approach, various subprograms are itemized in the income statement and are represented separately in individually identified revenue and expense categories. Various products might produce large or small amounts of revenue and thus generate large or small amounts of profit. This non-GAAP analysis allows managers to isolate solid or weaker performers in their product lines and to further consolidate these observations into an overall statement of the effectiveness of their product development. In the case of clinical activities, this approach can be used to identify activities that do or do not yield value or that have values with respect to each other. One might sort out different activities in an overall disease management program that are worth keeping or discarding, for example.

Finally, a term frequently used in medical management is *opportunity cost*. Opportunity costs generally refer to those costs forgone by not taking an action, by spending available

| Product | A | B | C | Total |
|---------|---|---|---|-------|
| **TABLE 6-5** | **Example of Activity-Based Cost Accounting** | | | |
| *Revenue* | | | | |
| Variable Revenue | $50 | $50 | $20 | $120 |
| *Expenses* | | | | |
| Variable Expense | $30 | $5 | $5 | $40 |
| Fixed Expense | $15 | $30 | $5 | $50 |
| **Profit (Loss)** | $5 | $15 | $10 | $30 |

monies on some other item or service, or by taking some alternative course of action. For example, the opportunity cost created when refurnishing an office can be expressed by the revenue lost by not using that same money to build an in-office lab or to buy X-ray equipment for a clinic.

### Accounting Skills Needed by Medical Managers

All of the accounting tools described are easily modeled on spreadsheets. The need for medical managers to develop the necessary skills to create financial models on spreadsheets cannot be overestimated. Using spreadsheets to create these models eases communication with other areas of the organization or the company that are involved in financing and approving the budgets for clinical programs.[20] For example, activity-based cost accounting might allow medical managers to isolate various programs under their control and to break out the components for analysis. Such an approach is also useful in medical facilities that track individual doctors, medical groups, or facility locations.[21]

An overall understanding of financial accounting and formal financial statements is important to comprehend the state of an organization or a company and the language of business. A working knowledge of managerial accounting is useful to communicate with people elsewhere in the organization. For example, medical managers must develop budgets that project anticipated costs for their organization. A medical manager who is not familiar with the various categories of cost in the budget and the ways in which these costs can be modeled on spreadsheets is at a clear disadvantage.

Other disadvantages of a lack of exposure to finance and accounting principles are more subtle. For example, medical directors often report that the assigned office overhead or the percentage of the organization's fixed expenses is high for their group. If the organization's *allocation strategy*, another concept in accounting for "internal cost transfers," focuses on overall salary rather than head count, a group with higher salaries could be penalized by having to absorb a disproportionately higher share of office overhead. Medical managers who shun the study of finance as too threatening or too boring might not pick up such detail, and their ability to obtain funds for future organizational expansion may be affected. Similarly, requests by medical managers to increase staffing in a quality improvement department are often met with skepticism because solid accounting measures or business models to justify the expansion are lacking. Developing financial and accounting skills, or acquiring staff who have these skills, is becoming critical to the success of quality management departments.

## Finance

Medical managers should be familiar with common financial terms and how these terms are used in an organization, particularly if they are seeking to become recognized as legitimate managers in a large organization. Financial concepts that medical managers need to understand are those involving the *cost of capital*, *discounted cash-flow analysis*, and *budgeting*.

### Cost of Capital

Long- and short-term financial management decisions may be less applicable to junior or even senior medical managers than to financial managers. Nevertheless, medical managers must understand the effect of the cost of their department on the overall finances of the organization. The organization's finance officers are interested in the "expected rate of return" of various efforts by the organization. However, the expected rate of return is particularly difficult to calculate and to communicate for medical initiatives that typically are not sold and that have only indirect relationships to changes in medical care costs. The effect of medical management activities often is not felt for many years, if at all, and the overall lack of certainty and precision complicates communication with financial managers who are trained to work with more precise terms.

Other communication difficulties may arise because medical managers do not comprehend the value of capital. For example, medical management staff often do not appreciate that money used to fund various projects has a value of its own—that is, the value that it might achieve if it were invested in something else, even a bank account. The amount represents the opportunity cost that was sacrificed by using the money in this way as opposed to some other way. Aggressive valuation techniques subtract this amount from the ultimate return from a program to determine *economic value added*.[22] Incorporating these financial concepts when requesting additional funding for clinical activities is important to make a successful case to senior management.[9]

### Discounted Cash Flow Analyses

Discounted cash flow analyses look at the time value of money. Briefly put, "money now is better than money later." For example, investing $100 at an interest rate of 8% will yield $108 in 1 year; being owed $108 next year is the equivalent of being paid $100 now. The formula Future Value (FV) = Present Value (PV) × (1 + Interest Rate) creates a relationship that converts future cash or benefit into present dollars, in *net present value* calculations.

Discounting future value in terms of present value in this way is frequently done in finance and is the accepted method used by financial officers to make those conversions. Familiarity with the correct use of this tool is important. Clinical managers often get into difficulty by trying to define more nebulous "quality gains" or "medical cost savings" in current economic terms. Incorrect use of the analysis or faulty conclusions can result.

### Budgeting
Working together on budgets is probably one of the most direct interactions that medical management staff has with financial staff. Senior managers unfamiliar with budgets frequently neglect the complicated, often tedious spreadsheets and accounting statements required by other departments and underestimate the importance of these documents to the rest of the organization. As a result, the authority to prepare and interpret these documents is often yielded to persons with less commitment to understanding and managing clinical activities.

Budgets are prepared differently in nearly every organization but typically follow structures that are similar to the structure of the income statement. Presented on a month-by-month basis and usually on spreadsheets, an entire year's expenses can be projected. The inability to follow a budget or to understand why individual budget categories are exceeded creates financing problems for senior management that, in turn, degrade medical managers' ability to function in an organization. Attention to budgets, while tedious, is a worthwhile exercise that should be undertaken by all medical managers, whether or not they are directly involved in the budgeting process.

## Other General Business Principles

Medical managers need a general understanding of how the business community works. Several concepts are extremely important to help them interact with others in the organization. These concepts include:

1.  Organizational planning and the planning process
2.  Project management
3.  Creation of business plans
4.  Preparation of pro forma financial statements
5.  Performance of sensitivity analyses
6.  An understanding of organizational psychology

### Organizational Planning and the Planning Process
Considerable resources are often dedicated to planning in health care organizations. The importance of this process cannot be overstated. Effective planning ultimately results in the creation of a detailed project management plan for the organization that defines specific activities.

Planners often start by formulating an overall view of the purpose of the organization, called the *mission statement*. This statement is designed to identify the key reason for the organization's existence and is often limited to one or two sentences. Planners may also create a *vision statement* for the organization that provides an overview of the organization's goals, often with a bias of describing how the organization will fare under idealized circumstances. After planners define the organization's mission and vision, they often develop high-level *goals*, which outline how the organization will attain its mission. A statement of goals typically contains 5 or 10 major elements, around which the business will focus in the coming year. Each goal has associated measurable *objectives* that must be met by a specified time to ensure that the goal is reached. Project management grids typically identify each objective and outline key tactical steps needed to achieve the objectives. Thus, from the high-level mission statement, the organization's planners can define goals for achieving that mission and specific objectives and tactics that will help to achieve the identified targets.

Managers also like to create SWOT charts that list numerically strengths, weaknesses, opportunities, and threats for the business or the planned activity. Working through these types of analyses in a group planning process often brings to light considerations that later become essential elements of the business planning process.

After planners have formulated goals and objectives, they typically move on to the detailed operational targets or achievable milestones that are listed in the management plan. Good managers usually name specific measures that indicate whether the plan is on track and record them regularly. *Lag measures* inform planners retrospectively as to whether their goals have been achieved. Examples are (1) records of net profits obtained after the corporation's books have been closed each month and (2) patient satisfaction survey results. *Lead indicators*, which inform managers whether the corporation is on track to meet a goal, are equally important. Examples are (1) patient flow measures (e.g., new patient visits) as a means of assuring new patient flows, and (2) average daily collections used to predict monthly earnings.

## Project Management

Project management becomes essential as the organization moves to assure that the desired flow of information and direction is maintained throughout the year. Poorly managed organizations frequently fail to crisply identify goals and objectives or spend considerable time in planning without achieving tangible results. To be successful, clinical quality managers need training in project management and the ability to carry out the planning sequence. Several accreditation organizations, such as the National Committee for Quality Assurance (NCQA), provide outlines for these types of planning processes as part of their required training. The leaders of these organizations have learned, as have many managers, that a well-thought-out and organized plan assures results when implemented effectively. Execution and results, not discussion or published articles, define success.

Good project management assures that all members of the initiative team understand their roles and responsibilities and know whether they are on track to execute the identified plan. Among the typical tasks of project management are identifying each key component of the project, identifying a person accountable to start the project, and setting an anticipated completion date. Simple grids, presented in spreadsheet form, can often be used in place of more expensive, formal project management programs, such as Microsoft Project.

## Creation of Business Plans

Successful business managers report that a key to their success is the ability to plan and to orchestrate a business initiative properly. Having a well-conceived business plan is frequently cited as a main factor for assuring that an initiative is executed. Business plans can be created through many approaches, most of which have been published in standard business planning textbooks. An effective business plan is disciplined and focused, combining various components of the financial analysis to make the business case for proceeding with the initiative.

The key elements of a business plan, each typically described in a few paragraphs, include the following:

1. An overview of the industry or company and a description of any products that are being produced or are under consideration

2. An evaluation of the current market, including the advantages of the proposed initiative over competitors' initiatives

3. A formal outline of the proposed initiative and the opportunities that it provides to the company

4. Market research that identifies the potential target market and the projected costs and revenues for the initiative

5. A formal design for implementing the initiative and a development schedule

6. An overall operations plan that uses standard project-management approaches

7. A profile of the accountable lead person and the credentials of the management and operations teams

8. An overview of the economics regarding the business and the initiative, including such areas as general profitability and sales potential

9. Anticipated risks and problems that could result in less-than-optimal outcomes

10. Financing arrangements and pro forma financial statements that outline return and costs over a period of several years

11. Estimated contracts, terms, agreements, and other items that must be negotiated

12. Exit strategy: the process for ending or discontinuing the program

The financial analysis, which need not be longer than five pages, may be presented in graphic or tabular form. Overall, the business plan should be a convincing statement that can be understood easily by a nonbusiness partner. A business plan typically projects a financial loss in the first year or two of development and a profit in subsequent years. The reasons for the projected losses in the initial years are typically scrutinized carefully by financial managers to assure that the losses will not persist.

### Preparation of Pro Forma Financial Statements

*Pro forma financial statements*, which are typically part of a business plan, detail the financial cost and expenses of a project for several time periods in the future.[23] These statements generally identify cost savings and expenses for a project in each of the coming three years, as well as overall profitability and ROI. Pro forma financial statements are used throughout the planning and financial process to give financial managers an overview of the long-term effectiveness of a project. They are particularly useful when a project has high start-up costs and thus may appear to be financially untenable.

### Performance of Sensitivity Analyses

In *sensitivity analysis*, which is often calculated using spreadsheets, the business project is modeled around a few initial key variables. The variables are then altered through a range of possible values, and the effect on outcomes is noted. Sensitivity analyses allow managers to determine the best- and worst-case outcomes of their undertaking with respect to numbers of participants, financial ROI, or other factors.

### An Understanding of Organizational Psychology

An important but often overlooked component in the business education of quality management professionals is the understanding of basic organizational psychology. This term refers to the complex interaction of individuals in an organization and how these interactions advance or interfere with the overall business direction of a firm. The related principles and strategies are described in detail in Chapter 4.

## Making the Business Case for Quality Management

Surprisingly, little has been written about how to develop the business case for quality management in a health plan.[24] Often, medical management presentations are not compelling, and medical directors and quality management professionals feel marginalized or isolated from the rest of the management staff. Further, the approach to understanding the concept of medical management varies with one's perspective (e.g., society, payer, provider, patient); how one might identify costs and benefits (e.g., intangible, direct, medical, indirect, nonmedical); and the type of analysis one performs to determine whether medical management is effective.[25] Methods used to indirectly create value estimates for other business types can also be investigated.[26]

An analysis of the economic value of quality management should take into account the following factors.

## Government Mandates

In the United States, the government has created a virtual mandate for quality management programs in health care by forcing large organizations to pay attention to the issue of medical quality. The government has mandated these programs directly and indirectly by specifying that external accrediting agencies be used. These external agencies withhold full accreditation unless certain quality programs and processes are in place, sometimes even specifying which ones are to be used. Such agencies include the CMS, the NCQA, the URAC, the Joint Commission, and local state departments of health and insurance, among others. This evolving "quality bureaucracy" has increased dramatically in size and complexity over the past several years. New programs are continually being added, existing programs are being expanded, and the linkages among the programs and various agencies and organizations are being forged at a pace that has been challenging for a single department in a managed care company or a hospital to coordinate and oversee.

## Demands by the Business Community

Recognizing the same issues, various payers in the business community (usually large employers) are also requiring or demanding participation in quality programs.

## Requirements for Quality Oversight

Because current requirements for medical management and quality oversight are extensive, clinical management departments typically need to manage multiple programs and, through their research, to identify programs that can be used to satisfy more than one criterion or standard at a time. Creating programs that have a competitive administrative overhead structure necessitates being frugal with resources and using individual initiatives to handle multiple demands.

## Demands of Business Partners

Various accounts or business partners may mandate the quality improvement activities of an organization. The need to comply with mandates is an effective argument for properly funding these activities, but it will not address the issue of whether resources are used most appropriately or efficiently by medical managers.

## Financial Effect

The financial effect of quality improvement activities on an organization is usually fairly small. Although the overall cost initially may seem high to financial managers, it can often be shown to be quite small on a PMPM basis across affected individuals in a health plan. An effective strategy might be to compare the costs of quality management in health care with those of similar efforts in other industries.

## Trade-Off Between a Higher Accreditation Standard and Lower Cost

The organization might develop several scenarios under which quality improvement programs could be increased or decreased. Decreasing these activities typically results in challenges from accreditation agencies, such as a reduction from an excellent to an accredited rating by the NCQA. Senior management will need to determine whether to commit to the highest level of quality or to risk and tolerate a lower accreditation standard in exchange for a decreased cost to the organization. Market forces play a key role in assigning values to these types of prioritizations.

## Results of Estimates Using Mathematical Tools

The benefits of quality management activities in mathematical terms have been estimated using tools such as the NCQA quality dividend calculator, which is available on the NCQA Website (http://www.ncqa.org/tabid/181/Default.aspx).

## Social Goals

The goal of quality can be more than financial. The mission of an organization, the desire to do the right thing, and the general pursuit of excellence are reasonable justifications for quality-related programs. Major employers are beginning to recognize the importance of employee satisfaction, productivity, and reduced absenteeism as goals in the delivery of health care.

Most health plan quality directors will eventually attempt to produce a comprehensive evaluation of quality management activities based on the points outlined. A comprehensive listing of the many demands made on an organization by various organizations creates a strong case for the existence of a single department to deal with them. Next, quality managers must show that compliance-related quality improvement activities are conducted as efficiently as possible by comparing benchmarks with organizations of similar size and business scope and by demonstrating that multiple requirements are addressed by each activity.

Justifying quality management activities at the level of an individual initiative often requires a different approach. Clinical initiatives frequently are multidimensional problems that have high variation and are nonlinear in scope. Clinical activities do not lend themselves to simple, linear approaches like the ROI calculations one might do for a simple loan or business proposal. They have complex cost functions that change over time, and there are no standing accounting methods to present them to senior management; that is, there are no GAAPs available to discuss the financial impact of medical management initiatives.[27,28]

Recently, as the total amount of money available for health care becomes increasingly limited, economists are working to determine the relative value of different interventions in the form of cost-effectiveness analysis. Developed in various ways, these efforts seek to combine both costs and clinical effectiveness in a single statistic or equation to estimate the impact or "bang for the buck" from various clinical activities. If one has only a million dollars to spend on all clinical programs, for example, the best allocation of scarce dollars can be guided by these methods.[29-35]

Although these factors make an analysis difficult, it should be undertaken in any event.

## Outcomes Categories

Quality management returns can be presented in economic terms using a variety of methods: financial, clinical, social, intangible, productivity based, and operational.[9]

### Financial

The benefit of a quality management initiative can be presented in terms of financial savings, for example, hard dollar savings, soft dollar savings, or imputed savings. *Hard dollar savings* are often the most difficult to demonstrate because a set amount of savings is predicted; for example, $1.50 saved for every $1.00 invested in an initiative. More typically, the benefit of an initiative is expressed in *soft dollar savings*, which are presented as a range in which the savings is likely to fall (say, between $0.94 per $1.00 invested, a negative ROI, and $3.00 per $1.00 invested, with a likelihood of about $1.50 in savings per $1.00 invested). These typical ranges are often difficult for senior managers to accept, and considerable effort is needed to demonstrate that the dollar savings is positive. *Imputed savings* are more readily demonstrated because they are compiled from evidence in the literature. Here, a clinical background is useful because the quality manager identifies the ROI from a multicenter, randomized, double-blind, placebo-controlled trial. For example, such a trial may show the ROI for influenza vaccine to be $16.00 per dose of vaccine administered. By proposing that an additional 5000 doses be administered through the hospital or plan program, the medical manager imputes that $80,000 in savings will accrue. Although convincing to a clinician, this evidence may be less so to a financial manager. The case can be strengthened by an analysis showing the change in influenza-related costs to the plan as well.

### Clinical

The rationale for conducting quality improvement activities can also be explained in terms of clinical improvement in care; however, clinical improvements are often difficult to describe in economic terms. For example, even though increasing the mammography rate is thought to reduce the progression to more complicated cancers and to increase the number of early cancers identified at the curative stage, its value for reducing medical care costs, or even saving individual lives, has not been established. The inability to establish a close link between the clinical activity and the cost savings makes moving to ROI logic difficult. Clinical improvement must be advanced on the basis of *willingness to pay*, an economic term used to describe the subjective estimation of valuation that accompanies making a purchase decision in the absence of a more rigorous accounting approach.[36] The lack of a clear path from clinical outcomes to the financial value of a clinical initiative makes budgeting difficult and puts senior management in the position of having to determine whether or not the clinical activity is worth the additional investment without a concrete method for doing so.[24,37]

*Social or Intangible*
Some reasons for undertaking quality management initiatives are unrelated to finances or to clinical matters and instead have social value. This category of evaluation in the business plan needs to be placed prominently in front of senior management. Intangible outcomes may include increased patient satisfaction, perception in the market that the institution is on the "leading edge" with the attached sales implications, and so on. Again, these benefits fall into the willingness to pay category.[36] Although it is important to evaluate the major dimensions of outcomes in medical management, we should not forget a long list of intangible elements of value that, while not easily measured, represent a real impact to clients.

Briefly, in this category we would answer the question, "If you spent $10 million on our programs and you saved $10 million in medical care costs, would you still do the program?" In other words, if the ROI was a break-even at 1.0, what elements would make you still consider the program?

Some of the elements in your answer should include the following.

**The Improvement of Sales**    Medical management is often viewed by the health plan sales team as an enhanced differentiator in health plan sales. Being seen as on the leading edge and in other ways presenting current programs is a clear market differentiator, even if these programs are seen as of modest economic value by skeptical elements of the internal team.

**Community Image**    In a related view, hospitals and health plans have a vested interest in enhancing the health of their members and the community. Clearly, medical management programs that emphasize wellness, the maintenance of good health, and similar goals are viewed by the community as a sign of good corporate citizenship. Sales and marketing staff frequently point to this as one of the values of these medical management programs.

**Human Resources Impact**    The development of an in-house medical management program is costly from a number of perspectives. This may allow considerable market power to sellers of these services, such as physician multispecialty medical practices and disease management companies that have built similarly functioning systems. First, the time to develop these programs represents a significant drag on management and internal staff as these programs are designed and built. This is particularly true for a specialty program requiring nurses with advanced skills in oncology or maternity, who may be hard to come by in a market in which there are widespread nursing shortages. This is an important consideration. Human resource development, including hiring staff, moving individuals physically from place to place, developing medical policy, and so on, is both costly and time consuming. Software support for medical management activities that are neither standard case management nor typical claims processing requires further modification, involving long delays as overworked information technology departments need to design, to test, and to implement programs. Finally, technical support to provide for the ongoing maintenance of a database containing current evidence-based guidelines and protocols is time consuming and costly. For all of these reasons, the sheer human capital cost of bringing programs online, even if conceptually simple in themselves, can be quite expensive. This, of course, is a decision for the individual institution, but there is a compelling logic to use a subcontractor with a great deal of experience in this area to support more complex functions.

**Provider Relations**    Medical management programs that are supportive to health plan physicians carry some positive public relations value in themselves. Well-practiced medicine compatible with evidence-based medicine guidelines is viewed positively by physicians, and infrastructure support, whether directly or indirectly in support of the "medical home" concept, can be presented to physicians as a positive effort on the part of the plan to make their job easier. Conversely, inaccurate or incomplete execution of these types of programs makes the health plan appear to be ineffective, out of touch, or incompetent to the practicing physician community.

**Future Savings**    Future savings provided by medical management are very difficult to quantify and are usually eliminated from the savings calculations. However, consider the long-term economic impact that might occur if all patients with diabetes properly take their medications and do not develop retinopathy, nephropathy, and neuropathy as complications. The long-term consequences of inadequate preventive medicine are well known and documented in the medical literature but, unfortunately, are poorly quantified from an economic perspective. Long-term economic gains can be clearly demonstrated in the primary and the secondary prevention of the major disease management categories that may be even greater in efforts to maintain wellness and a wellness culture within a business or health plan population.

**Accreditation–Compliance**    Various regulatory bodies and accreditation organizations view disease management and medical management as essential components in the ongoing business of the health plan. Full accreditation frequently requires attention to disease management and, increasingly, wellness efforts. The accreditation in itself has marketing impact with certain corporate business segments and delivery channels.

**Price Differential Effects**    Medical management programs targeting individuals within corporations or health plans have, as a secondary effect, the likely reduction in long-term health care costs. This in turn has the potential to reduce the short- and long-term trend and the pricing differential or profit potential accordingly delivered. Historically, community-based, physician-targeted programs improve care and lower costs for the whole community. Individual or member-based programs theoretically give a cost advantage to a health plan (because they only affect the plan's members) and might be preferred, as this attribute is emphasized to operational managers and senior management.

**Clinical Knowledge**    The ongoing development of medical management programs in general, and disease management and wellness in particular, creates positions within health plans that increase the overall clinical knowledge repository that is useful for other business functions, such as the development of accurate medical policy and corporate strategy concerning health policy in sales or government relations. Risk-management initiatives, the medical director's relationship with the medical community, and a variety of other, similar types of business-related activities are supported by the increased infrastructure and/or external expertise provided by carve-in or carve-out disease management programs.

Overall, the intangible values of medical management activities in general, and disease management and wellness programs in particular, come through a variety of the dimensions outlined. These should be included regularly in sales presentations and not omitted simply because they are unable to be easily quantified for highly analytical individuals. Most of the reasons resonate clearly at the chief executive officer (CEO)–chief operating officer and human resources level, given the absence of documented, directly linked ROI.

*Productivity Based*

There has been a recent upsurge in awareness and incorporation of productivity issues in outcomes measurement. "Absenteeism," "presenteeism," and general productivity have been advanced as important quality outcomes within the wellness community and by corporate sources. Understanding that the productivity impact of illness can contribute as much as three or four times the medical claims cost has precipitated a deep interest in the overall value of human health and "human capital" at both the employer and the individual levels.[38,39]

*Operational Methods*

The benefit of a quality management program can also be shown in terms of its ability to deliver the program elements. Although this approach might first be dismissed as purely a process rather than an outcome measure, the two have relevant points of overlap. In a disease management program, for example, the theory of the program may not be in doubt. Randomized, multicenter trials may have proven repeatedly that the elements of the program deliver value. For example, beta-blockers have been shown to help patients after a heart attack, and good diabetes control reduces long-term costs. What the program may need is the ability to deliver these elements to an entire population in a reasonable time, because taking several years to enroll a population, or to enroll only a fraction of the population, will not deliver value. Low or high operational performance in the implementation of a quality program or medical initiative is a quality indicator, because failure to implement the program will produce no results.[9]

In summary, quality managers must understand that the component pieces of quality management initiatives are often difficult to identify in financial terms but that a structured evaluation, as part of the business proposal value proposition, is necessary to allow the appreciation of value by those evaluating the activity.

## CASE STUDY • • •

### *Making the Business Case for a New Hospital Operating Unit*

As part of its QI efforts, a tertiary care pediatric children's hospital noted that it was not on par with best practices regarding the preoperative preparation of some of their critically ill children and those with chronic conditions. A proposal was made to create a Preanesthesia Consult Clinic (PACC). To present the material to senior management and to obtain buy-in with financial commitment, a business case and financial pro forma were created. The approach taken was to demonstrate simultaneous direct profit from the PACC and indirect savings through efficiency and quality effects from improved operating room (OR) management. Financial risk would be negligible, and the QI effort independently sustainable.

The PACC would both telephonically screen and physically evaluate patients with the purpose of assuring timely patient preparation and minimizing cancelled or forfeited OR times. While the majority of the screening work would be done as a virtual clinic, with contact via telephone, the PACC would also physically see (i.e., submit bills for), on average, 5 consults a day or 20 patients a week, for a billable amount of approximately $5000/week or $260,000/year.

For the leadership team, benefits included realization of direct revenues and real but somewhat less tangible improvement in operating efficiency and safety, including reduced waiting for OR cases to begin. Necessary preoperative work, such as obtaining consults and lab work, would be done ahead of time. It has been approximated that the cost of an OR delay is $10 per minute and the cost of a cancellation to be up to $1500 per hour. The PACC would be positioned to minimize cancellations and delays through a more efficient preadmission process. The case presented suggested that if even one 15-minute block of OR time could be better utilized each day, that would be a $150/day savings. Additionally, if even one cancellation of an hour-long case every other day could be avoided, it would translate to a weekly savings of $3750. This would result in total savings of $4500/week or at least $252,000/year. These were minimum assumptions, as internal studies of the OR demonstrated the rate of delays and cancellations to be higher than those noted. All were outlined in the formal plan.

The PACC would result in gross revenues for the hospital of $512,000/year. Expenses were mainly for staffing—the PACC needed to be staffed appropriately. The proposal planned for one full-time employee (FTE) registered nurse (RN; $90,000/year), one FTE licensed practical nurse ($50,000/year), two FTE nurse practitioners ($120,000/NP/year), and one 0.25 FTE anesthesiologist ($75,000/year) to run the PACC. Existing hospital facilities would be used, and initial start-up costs would thus not need to include office space, secretarial support, or additional costs. Start-up capital would be minimal, and the program could be terminated at the end of one year if results did not meet expectations.

Thus, the final business case for the leadership was that the costs for the PACC would be at approximately $455,000/year, offsetting the revenues described. With a budget of

$500,000/year, the PACC would be anticipated to cover its own costs and potentially even provide a minimal profit to the institution. The executive leadership approved the budget and the plan. The effective manner used to seek funding for quality improvement projects in this large institution created an improvement in the operating unit. By specifying a tight business pro forma and not relying on the intangible and unquantifiable quality outcomes, the team was successful in its approach to senior management. (See Table 6-6 for Pro Forma statement.)

TABLE 6-6    Pro Forma Financial Statement: Preanesthesia Consult Clinic

| Revenues | | Annualized Costs | |
|---|---|---|---|
| PACC Consultations— 20 consults per week | | $260,000 | |
| Efficiency Savings from historical data | | $252,000 | |
| | | Net Revenues | $512,000 |
| Expenses | | | |
| RN | 1 FTE | $90,000 | |
| LPN | 1 FTE | $50,000 | |
| NP | 1 FTE | $120,000 | |
| NP | 1 FTE | $120,000 | |
| Anesthesia MD | 0.25 FTE | $75,000 | |
| | | Net Expenses | $455,000 |
| | | Profit (Loss) | $57,000 |

# Pay-for-Performance (P4P) and Quality

Efforts in this decade by business, government, and health plans to control costs and to improve quality focus on the strategy of more richly rewarding physicians who deliver care at a higher level of quality. Pay-for-performance (P4P) strategies have been a continuous extension of the concept of incentive pay for physicians who, on average, perform below the expectations of payers and society at large.[40]

More recently, the industry has begun to sharply focus on true physician outcomes as opposed to process measures for improved reimbursement. Measures such as hospitalization rates and the percentage of patients with complete preventive medicine screens have found their way into a variety of P4P schemas.

An attendant concept to P4P is the "high-performance network," which has been advanced by a number of insurers and benefit management consultants. The proponents of these high-performance networks suggest that networks created by selecting only higher quality doctors should intrinsically be cheaper and better. Some develop a doctor quality index or cost-efficiency index and produce elaborate and impressive looking diagrams that seem to indicate that high-quality, high-cost doctors can deliver substantial improvements in cost and quality to purchasers of networks comprised of these physicians.[41] What remains a nagging issue in many of these special strategies is that there are very few solid examples of proof of concept. Most descriptions of special networks for incentive programs describe how it might be likely, reasonably, to derive cost savings and quality improvement from these systems, but very little solid evidence exists. There is even some concern that the value may not be there after all, despite the compelling intuitive logic.[41,42] The concern that high variability in claims data and individual practice composition might affect the year-over-year stability of an individual provider's quality rank also remains untested.

One of the most serious challenges to identifying high-quality physicians or networks is the issue of methodology. This can be broken down into a number of components.

First, there are no standardized methods for identifying what a high-quality physician is, particularly at the specialist level. Similarly, cost-effectiveness remains problematic because researchers are still struggling to identify appropriate levels of utilization and costs. Areas of low utilization and cost, for example, may just as likely represent underutilization of services as optimal utilization. The optimal level of utilization or performance is not easily determined across the very wide range noted around the country. Arbitrary set points for aggregate indices are highly challenging for most researchers to defend.

There are a number of approaches that have some common sense to undertaking them, such as paying physicians more for each patient for whom five major categories of diabetes, preventive medicine, and/or intervention occur. Clearly, perfection may be the enemy of the good in this case, as beginning to move the quality needle is a key point in the P4P set of programs.

A second major issue is the high levels of normal variation that clinicians encounter in the care of patients due to patient demographics, overall access to standards of care, illness burden, and genetics. Often, the number of patients who are treated by individual physicians, and even hospitals, may be too low to achieve the statistical significance to determine whether the hospital or physician represents either a "star" or an underperformer. The work of Barbara McNeil and team at Harvard has described how difficult the simple creation of appropriate statistics can be. Indeed, this team has openly wondered whether it is even possible to calculate statistics at the provider level that will identify them as high-performing physicians.[43,44]

The issues of statistics become particularly significant when payment is applied to provider selection. Frankly, it is difficult to understand why more legal challenges to P4P activities have not occurred, particularly when there is "economic credentialing" and physicians are threatened with exclusion from high-quality networks. The implication that someone who does not receive a high-performance award is necessarily a lower performer is one that does not sit well with those who do not receive such awards (which, under the schemas, may indeed represent a majority of physicians rather than a minority).

From a statistical perspective, high levels of variation also are noted in the longitudinal performance of providers at both the institutional and the individual levels. This is logically related to the necessary use of small numbers of data elements in the calculation of many of the statistics used and to the inherent variability of the medical care delivery system and patients themselves. This is a profound weakness in the logic behind special networks. Typically, physicians who are in the star stratum in 1 year may not be in subsequent years due to changes in patient population (e.g., the death of several very ill patients) or practice styles (e.g., the addition of a new partner). Physicians often correctly point to demographic and illness-varied differences in their patient populations that can result in this variation, as well as the normal variation in the way medical care is needed and delivered. Physicians are increasingly demanding security or risk adjustment in some meaningful form to accompany profiling efforts to eliminate this effect.[45]

It is clear that not paying attention to methodology can result in considerable stress. Identification by the Health Care Financing Administration (now the CMS) of high- and low-quality hospitals based on mortality rates serves as an example of a spectacular mistake in the past century. While our understanding of statistics has become more sophisticated and these types of errors no longer occur, subtleties remain problematic.

Another issue in the development of high-quality physicians and high-quality networks is that "risk follows premium." Many new and adaptive health care products initially showed decreased premium costs of high quality as they received an influx of healthy, early-to-doctor patients who do not have concerns about risks and covered services as a result of underlying illness. As time goes on and the products gain wider community support, increased numbers of ill patients result in antiselection pressures that normalize the results of the initial experience and suggest that initial results from the "cherry picking" that occurs in many new products are often not sustainable as the patient population enlarges to a significant number of individuals and high-risk populations.

Assuming that some generally agreed upon metric for quality could be found, another problem identified in seeking to collect high-quality doctors into select networks comes from the basic observation that physicians are unevenly distributed geographically with respect to the quality of their services. Often, clumps of doctors with a "desired" skill level or service occur in certain locations with the absence of doctors with these skills in others. Aside from the fact that there is no constant and universally accepted definition of high-quality doctors, the effect is the inability to provide a network with even geographic coverage. Almost from the beginning, exceptions are necessary to allow areas that do not have star doctors to permit network coverage under geographic dislocation studies at the health plan or employer level.

Many of the imperfections in a system for identifying and reimbursing high-quality physicians are problematic, particularly if these systems are presented in network brochures or the media. Not including all of the specialists in a very large teaching hospital causes concern where specialization is occurring on their part. Similarly, physicians included on the list of high-quality doctors who are well recognized by the medical community as not being of high quality undermine the credibility of the system. Type I (when you believe your hypothesis is true when it is not) and Type II (when you believe it is not true when it is) errors in any methodology are common and can hurt P4P initiatives as they are exploited in a competitive environment.

Health quality rewards administered can also become a major issue and occupy considerable administrative time of those managing the programs. Graded, continuous systems (rheostat) often result in arguments between physicians and the measurement team as to which level is achieved. More discontinuous methods (such as a series of switches or points) also result in arguments about the validity of that particular system. The use of claims data, self-reported data, or other sources of information in the grading system each present new challenges of interpretation and administration.

Much of the research on changing physician behavior suggests that methods are more effective when they target an individual physician at the point of care, as opposed to an organization as well. The locus of the analysis and the granularity of the assessments can have a significant impact on the likelihood of physician motivation and behavior change toward the desired effects.

Finally, one of the more subtle problems encountered in P4P systems occurs in the form of political backlash. Hospital CEOs will complain loudly that all of their departments do not have representative high-quality physicians as defined by a particular method. The reality of political pressures and the need to force every hospital into the category of high quality is a very real problem for administrators of these systems and frequently undermines the validity of the process.

Clearly, P4P programs for quality need to acknowledge the real issues in the definition and measurement of quality. A number of systematic and nonsystematic factors can significantly affect interpretation of results when payment is tied to a reward system for physicians. Flaws in the process of either identifying high quality or paying for it can significantly undermine the effort.

However, there is hope. Ongoing efforts to address the issues raised are beginning to emerge, particularly with the creation of electronic medical record systems, which can document physician performance and provide real-time feedback about areas targeted by P4P schema. Economics remains an important motivator of innovative solutions to pressures to change physician behavior.

## CASE STUDY ● ● ●

### *The Impact of P4P on the Delivery of Quality*

A large, multispecialty provider group in northern California used an existing chronic disease care management (CDCM) program to assist with the management of cholesterol for selected, specific high-risk patients. The program would allow reporting of measures that potentially would be used for P4P. Patients followed in the CDCM program had statistically significantly higher rates of low-density lipoprotein cholesterol (LDL-C) testing and goal attainment than patients followed in the routine manner of this group. The actual gain in revenue from the

CDCM is confidential; it is hypothesized to be approximately $28,000, assuming a $1 incentive per patient per month who meets the goal—and assuming that this multispecialty group was above the percentile slated to receive payments. The advantage of the CDCM for this group is that it utilized existing infrastructure and thus did not require start-up costs, which allows for the P4P monies to be considered as a potential source of revenue.

The ROI for this program is impossible to calculate as there were no real extraneous costs to the program for the multispecialty group. For this program to be implemented de novo, we might cautiously estimate the time of approximately 0.5 FTE at the RN level (about $45,000/year). Therefore, a program that generates revenue for the above-mentioned multispecialty group ends up generating a loss in another practice setting.

*Adapted from:* Cutler TW, Palmieri J, Khalsa M, Stebbins M. Evaluation of the relationship between a chronic disease care management program and California pay-for-performance diabetes care cholesterol measures in one medical group. *J Manag Care Pharm.* 2007;13(7): 578–588.

In this chapter we have also discussed the time frame of an ROI. In specific disease states, the ROI (or cost savings) can be appreciated in a short time frame (e.g., influenza vaccinations for a seasonal disease process) or over a much longer time frame (e.g., the effect of LDL-C levels on morbidity and mortality). With a largely transient and migratory pattern of patients, the effectiveness and financial case of P4P programs from the perspective of the administering organization must be considered. In the previous case study, the potential payment of $28,000 to the multispecialty group was only for approximately a fraction of the group. Would it be in the administering organization's financial interest to make a payment of $50,000 to this group if it was able to achieve target goal thresholds on all potential patients? Additionally, this cost to the administering organization is only for incentive payments to one multispecialty group! What of the other groups that receive payments for being above the goal threshold? The ROI to the practice may be different than the ROI to the sponsoring organization or employer, who may see P4P costs as paying for something the physicians are supposed to be doing anyway. The costs can be staggering, and it is incumbent upon the administering organizations that develop P4P programs to ensure that they have an adequate ROI. One could argue that the money saved may not be realized due to patients moving from one region to another, especially for a disease process such as one affected by cholesterol levels.

Thus, on many levels, this brief case study shows the inherent difficulties and subtle flows of money that make the ROI calculations very pertinent based on who is paying and who is receiving the incentive payments.

## Future Trends

The future of patient safety and quality improvement vis-à-vis a financial perspective will continue to evolve, especially as the government and the private sectors realize that ballooning health care expenditures contribute substantially to the slow growth of our economy. Whatever the future may bring with regard to varying payment schemes and incentive structures, the fundamentals of this chapter on economics and the role of the quality and safety manager in this arena will remain crucial to one's ability to maneuver in whatever the future may hold.

# References

1. Corrigan J, Greiner A, Erickson S. *Fostering Rapid Advances in Health Care: Learning from Systems Demonstrations.* Washington, DC: The National Academies Press; 2002.
2. Kohn L, Corrigan J, Donaldson M. *To Err Is Human: Building a Safer Health System.* Washington, DC: National Academies Press; 1999:1–13.
3. National Academy of Sciences. *Priority Areas for National Action: Transforming Health Care Quality* (Report). Washington, DC: National Academies Press; 2003.
4. Gold M, Siegel J, Russel L, Weinstein M. *Cost Effectiveness in Health and Medicine. Report of the U.S. Public Health Service Panel on Cost Effectiveness in Health and Medicine.* New York/Oxford: Oxford University Press; 1996.
5. Berwick D. *Curing Health Care. New Strategies for Quality Improvement.* San Francisco: Jossey-Bass; 1990.
6. Drummond M, McGuire A. *Economic Evaluation in Health Care. Merging Theory with Practice.* Oxford, UK: Oxford University Press; 2001.
7. Drummond M, O'Brien B, Stoddart G, Torrance G. *Methods for the Evaluation of Health Care Programmes,* 2nd ed. New York/Oxford: Oxford Medical Publications; 1998.
8. Millenson M. *America's Health Care Challenge: Rising Costs.* Washington, DC: American Association of Health Plans; 2002.
9. Leatherman S, Berwick D, Iles D, et al. The business case for quality: Case studies and an analysis. *Health Aff.* 2003;22(2):17–30.
10. Lindahl E. On Keynes' "economic system." *Economic Rec.* 1954;30:19–32, 159–171.
11. Dornbursch R, Fischer S. *Macroeconomics,* 5th ed. New York: McGraw Hill; 1990.
12. Jacobs P. *The Economics of Health and Medical Care.* Gaithersburg, MD: Aspen Publishers, 1996.
13. Scherer FM, Ross D. *Industrial Market Structure and Economic Performance,* 3rd ed. Dallas, TX: Houghton Mifflin; 1990.
14. Mansfield E. *Economics,* 6th ed. New York: WW Norton; 1989.
15. Wessels WJ. *Economics,* 2nd ed. New York: Barron's Educational Series; 1993.
16. Taylor T. *Economics (Part I and Part II).* Audio Tape Course. Chantilly, VA: The Learning Company; 1996.
17. Phelps C. *Health Economics.* New York: Addison Wesley; 1997.
18. Santerre R, Neun S. *Health Economics: Theories, Insights, and Industry Studies.* Chicago, IL: Irwin; 1996.
19. Academy for Healthcare Management. *Health Plan Finance and Risk Management* (Booklet). Atlanta, GA: Author; 1999.
20. Kaplan R, Cooper R. *Cost and Effect: Using Integrated Cost Systems to Drive Profitability and Performance.* Cambridge, MA: Harvard Business School Press; 1998.
21. Baker J. *Activity-Based Costing and Activity-Based Management for Health Care.* Gaithersburg, MD: Aspen Publishers; 1998.
22. Hubbell W. Combining economic value added and activity based management. *J Cost Manage.* 1996;10(1):18–29.
23. Gladowski P, Fetterolf D, Beals S, et al. Analysis of a large cohort of HMO patients with congestive heart failure. *Am J Med Qual.* 2003;18(2):73–81.

24. Fetterolf D. Commentary: Presenting the value of medical quality to nonclinical senior management and boards of directors. *Am J Med Qual.* 2003;18(1):10–14.
25. Eisenberg J. Clinical economics. A guide to the economic analysis of clinical practices. *JAMA.* 1989;262(20):2879–2886.
26. Luehrman T. What's it worth? A general manager's guide to valuation. *Harv Bus Rev.* 1997;75(3):132–142.
27. National Committee on Quality Assurance. NCQA Online Tool Demonstrates How Better Health Care Costs Less. http://www.ncqa.org/tabid/589/Default.aspx. Accessed October 15, 2008.
28. Plocher D, Brody R. Disease management and return on investment. In: Kongstvedt P, Plocher D, eds. *Best Practices in Medical Management.* Gaithersburg, MD: Aspen Publishers; 1998:397–406.
29. Blissenbach H. Use of cost consequence models in managed care. *Pharmacotherapy.* 1995;15(5):59s–61s.
30. Clancy C, Kamerow D. Evidence-based medicine meets cost-effectiveness analysis. *JAMA.* 1996;276(4):329–330.
31. Robert S, Galvin R. The business case for quality: Developing a business case for quality will require a deliberate approach, with all economic parties at the table. *Health Aff.* 2001; 20(6):57–58.
32. Haddix A, Teutsch S, Shaffer P, et al. *Prevention Effectiveness: A Guide to Decision Analysis and Economic Evaluation.* New York/Oxford: Oxford University Press; 1996.
33. Litvak E, Long M, Schwartz S. Cost-effectiveness analysis under managed care: Not yet ready for prime time? *Am J Manag Care.* 2000;6(2):254–256.
34. Torrance G. Preferences for health outcomes and cost-utility analysis. *Am J Manag Care.* 1997;3 suppl:S8–S20.
35. Weinstein M, Siegel J, Gold MR, et al. Recommendations of the panel on cost-effectiveness in health and medicine. *JAMA.* 1996;276(15):1253–1258.
36. Gafni A. Willingness to pay in the context of an economic evaluation of healthcare programs: Theory and practice. *Am J Manag Care.* 1997;3 suppl:S21–S32.
37. Fetterolf D, West R. The business case for quality: Combining medical literature research with health plan data to establish value for non-clinical managers. *Am J Med Qual.* 2004;19(2):48–55.
38. Loeppke R, Hymel P. Good health is good business. *J Occup Environ Med.* 2006;48(5):533–537.
39. Loeppke R, Taitel M, Richling D, et al. Health and productivity as a business strategy. *J Occup Environ Med.* 2007;49(7):712–717.
40. McGlynn E, Asch S, Adams J, et al. The quality of health care delivered to adults in the U.S. *N Engl J Med.* 2003;348(26):2635–2648.
41. Kazel R. Are HMOs dead? Or just on life support? *AMNews.* April 18, 2005:1.
42. Clickman S, Ou F, DeLong E, et al. Pay-for-performance, quality of care, and outcomes in myocardial infarction. *JAMA.* 2007;297:2272–2280.
43. McNeil B. Shattuck lecture: Hidden barriers to improvement in the quality of care. *N Engl J Med.* 2001;345(22):1612–1620.
44. Shahian D, Normand S, Torchiana D, et al. Cardiac surgery report cards: Comprehensive review and statistical critique. *Ann Thorac Surg.* 2001;72:2155–2168.
45. Iezzoni L. *Risk Adjustment for Measuring Healthcare Outcomes.* Chicago: Health Administrative Press; 1997.

## Additional Resources–Further Reading

George A, Schultz J. Regulation, incentives, and the production of quality. *Am J Med Qual.* 2007;22(4):265–272.

Birkmeyer J. Potential benefits of the new Leapfrog standards: Effect of process and outcomes measures. *Surgery.* 2004;135(6):569–575.

Birkmeyer J, Siewers A, Finlayson E, et al. Hospital volume and surgical mortality in the United States. *N Engl J Med.* 2002;346(15):1128–1137.

Birkmeyer J, Stukel T, Siewers A, et al. Surgeon volume and operative mortality in the United States. *N Engl J Med.* 2003;349:2117–2127.

Coddington D. *Making Integrated Health Care Work.* Englewood, CO: Center for Research in Ambulatory Health Care Administration; 1996.

The Commonwealth Fund. Measuring Provider Efficiency, Version 1.0: A Collaborative, Multi-Stakeholder Effort. http://www.commonwealthfund.org/publications/publications_show.htm?doc_id=257206. Accessed October 15, 2008.

Donabedian A. *Explorations in Quality Assessment and Monitoring. Vol II. The Criteria and Standards of Quality.* Ann Arbor, MI: Health Administration Press; 1982.

Epstein A, Lee T, Hamel M. Paying physicians for high-quality care. *N Engl J Med.* 2004;350(4):406–410.

Fetterolf D. Costs from a Third Party Payor Perspective. In: *Quality and Cost in Neurological Surgery.* Linskey ME, Rutigliano, eds. Philadelphia, PA: Lippincott Williams and Wilkins; 2001.

Fetterolf D, Jennings S, Moorhead T, May J. *Outcomes Guidelines Report.* Washington, DC: Disease Management Association of America; 2006.

Fetterolf D, Jennings S, Norman G, Moorhead T, May J. *Outcomes Guidelines Report.* Vol II. Washington, DC: Disease Management Association of America; 2007.

Fetterolf D, Sidorov J. *Disease Management Program Evaluation Guide.* Washington, DC: Disease Management Association of America; 2004.

Langley P. Is cost effectiveness modeling useful? *Am J Manag Care.* 2000;6(2):250–251.

McCulloch D. Managing diabetes for improved health and economic outcomes. *Am J Manag Care.* 2000;6(21 suppl):S1089–S1095.

McLaughlin CP, Kaluzny AD, eds. *Continuous Quality Improvement in Healthcare,* 3rd ed. Sudbury, MA: Jones and Bartlett; 2006.

Montgomery D. *Introduction to Statistical Quality Control,* 3rd ed. New York: John Wiley and Sons; 1997.

National Committee for Quality Assurance. HEDIS and Quality Measurement. http://www.ncqa.org/tabid/59/Default.aspx. Accessed October 15, 2008.

Reiter K, Kilpatrick K, Green S, et al. How to develop a business case for quality. *Int J Qual Health Care.* 2007;19(1):50–55.

Santerre RE, Neun SP. *Health Economics: Theories, Insights, and Industry Studies.* Chicago: Irwin; 1996.

Walton M. *The Deming Management Method.* New York: Perigee Books; 1986.

# Chapter 7

# Utilization Management

*Arthur L. Pelberg, MD, MPA*

## Executive Summary

*Utilization management* (UM) is the mix of clinical, administrative, and financial methods used to evaluate the appropriateness, the processes, the facilities, and the providers of care that are applied to an individual and a total population of patients. The evaluation approach typically uses evidence-based guidelines to make its decisions.

The underlying reasons for doing UM is to make sure that health care is delivered in the most efficient and effective manner for the patient and the population, where such activities directly impact the quality of outcomes. This contrasts with the older concept of utilization review that was performed to evaluate the cost of care. Intrinsic to utilization review is a structured program and methodology that incorporates indicators, monitors, and benchmarks to determine the outcomes of the UM process. Previously, the responsibilities of UM and quality management were very distinct, but more recently they have begun overlapping.

### Learning Objectives

Upon completion of this chapter, readers should be able to:

- describe the history and significant milestones in UM;
- discuss processes and methods of UM;
- discuss organizational design in the context of challenges to implementing UM;
- evaluate outcomes and the return on investment for UM; and
- describe the regulatory, accreditation, and oversight programs for UM.

## History

In the early 19th century, American medicine was disorganized and of poor quality. This caused a confederation of state and local societies to form the American Medical Association (AMA) in 1847. The AMA funded Abraham Flexner to create a report to the Carnegie Foundation that documented the deplorable state of the nation's medical schools and major hospitals.[1] Shortly thereafter, in 1914, Codman[2] recommended that each physician and hospital should be accountable for the outcomes of their patients (quality and utilization). This influenced the American College of Surgeons to establish its Hospital Standardization Program in 1917.[3] Included in the 1917 minimum standards program were:[3]

1. Organizing hospital medical staffs

2. Limiting staff to well-educated, competent, and licensed physicians

3. Framing rules and regulations to ensure regular staff meetings and clinical review

4. Keeping medical records that included the history, physical examination, and laboratory results

5. Establishing supervised diagnostic and treatment facilities

In 1952 the American College of Physicians, the American Hospital Association, and the Canadian Medical Association joined the American College of Surgeons to form the Joint Commission on Accreditation of Hospitals,[3] which mandated peer review. In 1965, the Congress passed Title XVIII of the Social Security Act, which enacted certain Conditions of Participation in Medicare that included utilization review.[4] In 1972, the Professional Standards Review Organization (PSRO) came into existence through an amendment to the Social Security Act. The PSRO was responsible to promote efficiency and to try to eliminate unnecessary hospital utilization; their emphasis was cost containment over quality.[5] In 1982, the PSRO was replaced by the Peer Review Organization (PRO), which was mandated to validate DRG coding, to reduce unnecessary hospital admissions and operations, and to improve the quality of care in the hospital.[6] The PRO program was subsequently renamed the Quality Improvement Organization (QIO) in 2002. The QIO is currently viewed as the major organization that will improve quality and efficiency of health care for Medicare beneficiaries. This has moved the QIO more toward quality oversight and away from a utilization focus.

## Critical Components of Utilization Management Systems

In order for UM programs to be successful, several critical factors must be in place, as described below.[7]

- Utilization data and information that can be easily compared between providers, patients, payers, and other stakeholders (e.g., the Pennsylvania Health Care Cost Containment Council information).

- Continued improvement in UM processes to keep pace with the complex care and new technology being used for credentialing.

- UM programs need to utilize up-to-date technology that does not duplicate the administrative burden of providers and patients.

- Safeguards to protect individual patient data and information as identified in the Health Insurance Portability and Accountability Act (HIPAA) and other regulations.

- UM programs must utilize evidence-based medicine, patient and provider satisfaction measures, cost of operations, and clinical outcomes of patients in determining the appropriateness and the success of UM efforts.

- Determinations must be reliable, consistent, and follow the policy of the UM program. The UM program must be responsive to patients and providers through a grievance and appeals program, quality monitoring system, and trending of the decisions of care (especially, denials of care).

- UM must occur without delaying care. There needs to be a process in place that reviews alternatives of care, placement of care, and providers of care in a timely fashion. In addition, the UM process must follow the coverage and benefit that is provided to the patient.

## The Utilization Management Process

This process includes interventions that take place before, during, and after a clinical event occurs. The process that occurs before the clinical event is called *prior authorization* or *precertification*. While the clinical event is happening, the process is called *concurrent review*; if the patient is in a facility, it will also include discharge planning. After the clinical event has occurred, the process is called *retrospective review* or *retro-review*. The UM process should be as nonintrusive to the delivery of care as possible, and be able to stop inappropriate care before it does harm.

## The Nine Tasks Key to Effective Utilization Management

There are nine key tasks that help UM to be consistent and relevant, to integrate into the organization, and to legitimatize the process among clinicians, patients, and other stakeholders.

### 1. Determine Priority Areas

These may be related to the use of health care resources, quality outcomes, regulatory compliance, and overall financial health of the health care organization. For many health care organizations, the majority of their revenue is spent on clinical care. The right questions will improve the clinical and the financial health of the organization.

### 2. Identify Needed Information and Critical Stakeholders

Data are required to guide the UM processes. The data must be accurate, timely, relevant, and easily collectable at a reasonable cost. The methodology of using the data must be transparent and appropriate. Stakeholder buy-in from senior management, providers, and patients is key to successful UM.

## 3. Establish Appropriate Benchmarks

Benchmarks must be chosen that will identify desired levels of performance. Benchmarks can represent the process or outcome of care. When evidence-based medicine does not have an appropriate benchmark for the study, an expert panel of clinicians may suggest a standard. Benchmarks may be internally or externally generated.

## 4. Design, Data Collection, and Data Management Procedures

There is presently no accepted methodology for UM studies. The NCQA has identified a generic improvement activity form that may be used by UM plans.[8] Appropriate determination of the sample size and procedure and the types of data to be used (administrative or clinical) are critical when evaluating performance for UM.

## 5. Implement Data Collection and Management Procedures

This includes the allocation of human and financial resources for UM. It is important to have policies and procedures in place to determine how the data collection and evaluation will occur. Policies and procedures must also be consistent and uniform across patients, providers, organizations, and other stakeholders. The cost of data collection must be evaluated.

## 6. Evaluate the Data and Present Results

There should be a common methodology and statistical analysis used in interpreting the data. Results must be presented in a fashion that recognizes speculation and ensures that the methodology and the statistical analysis of the study have been transparent and that the results can be attributed to the intervention.

## 7. Develop Guidelines, Policies, and Procedures

Once an area for improvement in structure, process, and/or outcome is identified, new guidelines must be developed by the organization. This change process should be managed by the organization and include key stakeholders (e.g., clinicians) affected by the change.

## 8. Implement Guidelines, Policies, and Procedures

System change can occur only if UM guidelines, policies, and procedures are implemented, followed, and re-evaluated on a regular basis.

## 9. Continuously Review the Task List

Each of the nine tasks identified should be reviewed on a regular basis by the people or the body responsible for UM in the organization in order to build a culture of constant improvement.

# Processes, Procedures, and Timing of Utilization Management

The UM plan usually contains operational procedures that are related to prior authorization, concurrent review, and retrospective review. While each of these can be applied a little differently by each entity doing the UM programs, there are standard procedures and reasonings behind each of the three processes.

## Prior Authorization or Precertification

The first process is prior authorization or precertification, which is performed before a clinical intervention takes place. The purpose of this process is to make sure the clinical intervention is appropriate and takes place in the right setting and time, and the clinician has the expertise to do the clinical intervention. All these criteria should be measured on the basis of evidence-based medicine for that particular condition. Milliman[9] and other vendors have developed criteria for prior authorization. Prior authorization can also be used as a vital communication link within a health care organization by gathering information and by distributing it to other parts of the organization that will help the patient have a better outcome. An example of this is a patient who is going in for a hip replacement. Once prior authorization information is received, it is transferred to a nurse who can call the patient to determine the individual's needs for rehabilitation (e.g., can the patient go home with appropriate support, does the patient need a placement in a rehabilitation facility). The nurse can also set up a satisfaction survey that will follow the patient after the episode of care is completed. This can include an SF-12 (a measure of perceived physiologic status and satisfaction before the procedure takes place and after the procedure is completed).

If the organization doing the prior authorization is also a payer of claims, the notification and approval will be sent to the finance area to make sure funds are available to pay the providers of the intervention. The prior authorization process will also notify other components of the UM program (including concurrent review and retrospective review) to ensure they are performed in a timely and appropriate manner.

## Concurrent Review and Discharge Planning

Concurrent review is the management of resources by evaluating the necessity, appropriateness, and efficiency of the use of medical services, procedures, and levels of care while a patient is in a facility. This usually occurs or takes place for urgent or elective acute hospital admissions. The purpose of concurrent review is to deliver efficient, effective health care; to reduce the occurrence of over-, under-, or misuse of inpatient services; and to promote the best outcome and patient safety during an inpatient stay. As with the prior authorization process, concurrent review is connected to other processes of care including quality monitoring of the patient's hospital stay, coordinating with discharge planning, and identifying appropriate next levels of care. Concurrent review also helps identify patients who may benefit from disease and/or case management and transfers data to finance for appropriate reimbursement. Criteria for concurrent review can vary by the organization performing the service, as long as it follows the principles of evidence-based medicine. Two recognized sources of criteria for concurrent review are Milliman Care Guidelines[9] and Qualis Health-McKesson's InterQual Criteria.[10]

*Discharge planning* is the process of arranging for the next level of care for patients as they are ready to leave the facility and may be considered part of the concurrent review process. Discharge planning is initiated when patients are first admitted to the hospital and takes into consideration the medical conditions, social and environmental concerns, financial status, and other variables to make certain that the patients receive the appropriate placement and services once they leave the facility. Discharge planning is usually a team effort involving nurses, social workers, primary and specialty physicians, and the patient or patient advocate.

## Retrospective Review

Retrospective review is the process of reviewing health care interventions and charges after the care has been delivered and the bill is submitted. Retrospective review determines whether the care was appropriate and provided at the most efficient and effective level with the best outcomes. It also determines if the bill was coded correctly according to CPT, CMS, ICD-9, or other guidelines. Retrospective review can be used to collect data on quality and utilization by physicians, health care organizations, and other providers of care.

## Interrater Reliability

Whenever a UM process has the potential to be evaluated by different reviewers, an *interrater reliability assessment* is required. Interrater reliability assessment is defined as the process of monitoring and evaluating clinical reviewers' understanding of medical review criteria and the consistency with which different reviewers apply the same criteria in making decisions. This important step is needed to certify that the review process decisions are made in a consistent manner according to evidence-based medicine criteria. Interrater reliability is usually assessed on a quarterly or semi-annual basis. Reviewers whose decisions are not consistent with the criteria are usually re-educated and retested.

## Measuring the Effectiveness of UM Programs

Generally, the effectiveness of UM programs is measured in financial terms, dollar savings, or ROI. Some programs will merge quality and utilization programs and measure their effectiveness by using a balanced scorecard approach. The effectiveness of UM should at least be based on the following:

1. Evidenced-based criteria
2. Reliable, accurate, and defensible data that has been validated
3. Appropriate clinical expert review
4. Transparent methodology of effectiveness calculations

There are always challenges in the calculation of effectiveness of UM. When looking at the results, one must consider the following potential problems:

1.  The sample size may be small or not appropriate for comparison.

2.  The sample population may be different by demographics, severity, or culture.

3.  There are no standardized methodologies across health care organizations on how to calculate ROI.

There has been some controversy over the value of UM. Several organizations have identified the cost of conducting UM as greater than the savings obtained from the process. As identified above, UM should be part of a group of interventions to decrease overuse, underuse, and misuse of health care and to improve individual and population outcomes. There should be a system in place that can identify patient safety issues that have been avoided by doing concurrent review in the hospital or identification of a quality problem that was reported before it became a major issue. The UM process may also enhance the patient experience with the health care system because of discharge planning and follow-up when the patient is out of the hospital. This could be represented in improved satisfaction survey results by the patient and the providers.

Table 7-1 is an example of a calculation used by a health care organization to evaluate its return for doing UM.

### TABLE 7-1  Concurrent Review (CR) Calculation

Claims data are identified for patients admitted to the hospital 6 months before the CR process is put in place. Another cohort is taken for 6 months after the CR process has been implemented. The patient samples are sorted by diagnosis and severity of illness to confirm that two similar populations are being compared. Then, criteria are reported by bed days/1000, average length of stay (ALOS) by diagnosis and population cohorts, average cost per discharge before and after CR, admission rate/1000, and readmission rate/1000. Other criteria may be used, depending on the interest of the organization. The difference between the pre- and post-CR process is calculated, and a unit cost for each hospital day is applied to give the total dollar amount of savings. The cost of the CR process is then added into the accounting process. This calculation can give a relative return on investment for the CR process. The example may look like the following:

| Criteria | Pre-CR | Post-CR | Delta |
|---|---|---|---|
| Admits/1000 | 70 | 45 | 25 |
| Bed days/1000 | 315 | 157.5 | 157.5 |
| ALOS | 4.5 | 3.5 | 1.0 |

The results show 157.5 bed days/1000 were avoided using CR. Each bed day cost $1385, resulting in savings of $218,138. The cost of the CR process was $25,000 for the same time period. The ROI for the CR process is 8.7:1 ($218,138/$25,000).

## Risk Management and Safety

*Risk management*, in its most general sense, can be defined as identifying circumstances that put patients or an organization at risk for adverse outcomes and putting into operation methods that avoid, prevent, and control the risks. In recent years, risk management, UM, quality management, and patient safety have had overlapping functions. An example of risk management in organizational terms is avoiding the use of a code cart that has not been restocked properly. For an individual patient, it may be confirming that all the protocols are followed when giving intravenous medications to the patient.

Risk management was adopted by hospitals when the Joint Commission added sentinel event monitoring to the accreditation process in the mid-1990s.[11] This coincided with a time when there were many problems in malpractice coverage that caused risk to be a potential problem for hospitals and health care organizations. (Further details on medical errors and adverse events are provided in Chapter 3.)

## Organizational Design of Utilization Management

Typically, the person responsible for the UM program is a health care professional with several years experience in the field of health care utilization, quality, risk management, and/or safety. A simple structure for an organization to use in setting up their program is shown in Figure 7-1.

It is imperative for the UM program to have clinical input from practitioners who must comply with the UM program. Some organizations have outside clinicians (who are not responsible to practice under the UM plan) help evaluate the validity and the appropriateness of the UM plan. This is usually done through a UM committee or a practitioner advisory committee. The functions of the committee are described in Table 7-2.

A senior clinician should lead the UM committee, and the committee should include several practicing physicians from different specialties and primary care. Committee meetings should be held on a regular schedule with support staff to help with the administrative aspects of the committee, such as keeping meeting minutes. The health care organization may also designate senior administrative leaders to serve on the committee. The committee should report to the decision makers in the health care organization.

## Disease Management

*Disease management* (DM) is defined as a system of coordinated health care interventions and communications for populations with conditions in which patient self-care efforts can significantly improve health care outcomes. The following are characteristics specific to disease management, and emphasize prevention of exacerbations and complications by the application of evidence-based medicine approaches.

- Support of the physician or practitioner–patient relationship and plan of care
- Stratification of patients by risk level

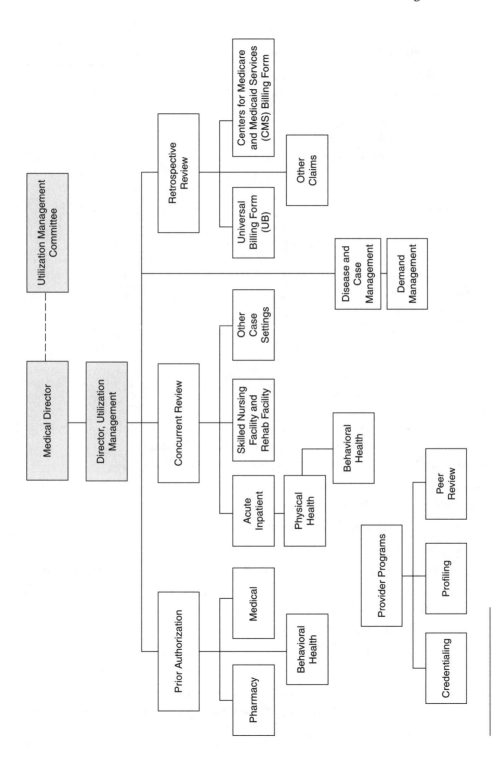

**Figure 7-1** Utilization Management: Model Organizational Structure

TABLE 7-2   Functions of a UM Committee

1. Design and development or planning
   a. Program structural design
   b. Identify opportunities to improve
   c. Identify performance indicators and metrics
   d. Identify organizational resources
   e. Align with organizational strategic plan

2. Monitoring the review activity
   a. Review progress of initiatives
   b. Develop senior leadership reports
   c. Track accreditation preparation

3. Communication with appropriate internal and external stakeholders
   a. Resource utilization progress
   b. Program impact to workforce and senior leadership
   c. Hold meetings to present results
   d. Recognize and reward efforts

4. Program evaluation
   a. Develop UM program evaluation measures
   b. Ensure accountability for program goals and objectives
   c. Present impact report

- Evaluation of clinical, humanistic, and economic outcomes on an ongoing basis with the goal of improving overall health for the individual
- An intended outcome of better patient self-management over time

DM programs differ according to the health care organization implementing the program; however, there are six components that a full-service DM program must have:

1. Population identification processes

2. Evidence-based practice guidelines

3. Collaborative practice models that include physician and support service providers

4. Patient self-management education including primary prevention, behavior modification, and compliance evaluation

5. Process and outcomes measurement evaluation and management

6. Routine reporting–feedback loop including communication with the patient, the physician, and other identified stakeholders under HIPAA regulations

The telephone is the most common communication mechanism between patients and the DM program, although some advanced programs use Web-based communication and text messaging to cell phones and other devices to contact patients. The return on investment for DM programs is just beginning to be standardized. DMAA: Care Continuum Alliance (formerly known as the Disease Management Association of America), National Committee on Quality Assurance (NCQA), and other organizations are developing standard methodological systems to calculate the ROI.

The most common DM programs for commercial populations are diabetes mellitus, congestive heart failure, asthma, cardiovascular disease, low back pain, and depression. There are movements in DM to cluster related diagnoses and chronic conditions together to create a more comprehensive program. Clusters may include asthma and COPD, hypertension and coronary artery disease, diabetes, congestive heart failure, and hyperlipidemia. DM programs should be built for the population being served by a careful analysis of the diseases that the population has been diagnosed with and the drivers of cost and quality for that population. This process of evaluation should be ongoing to identify and to adjust for changes in the demographics and use of health care so that new programs can be implemented.

## Case Management

*Case management* is defined as centralizing the planning, arranging, and follow-up of a member's specific health services in order to manage utilization, effectiveness, cost, and quality of health care. Case management is used to monitor and to coordinate medical and other services rendered to members—special populations who have specific diagnoses or require high-cost or intensive services. The process of case management coordinates designated components of health care, such as appropriate referral to consultants, specialists, hospitals, and ancillary providers and services. It will also help the patient with social and environmental concerns that may hinder or delay improvement in the medical condition. Case management helps the patient navigate through complex systems or different organizations and avoid fragmentation or misutilization of services. Case management works at the individual patient level and communicates frequently with the patient and the providers of care.

Key components of a case management program include the following:

1.  Screening and identification of conditions, populations, individual patients, and disease states for early detection of health problems.

2.  Identifying and implementing effective interventions for individuals using evidence-based medicine and removing social–environmental barriers to care.

3.  Promoting and coordinating a collaborative team approach across various disciplines and levels of care.

4.  Coordinating continuity of care through the course of the disease or condition to attain the best possible clinical outcome and improve quality of life.

5.  Coordinating support and education for the patient, patient's family, and others involved in the patient's care to improve and sustain self-management behaviors and quality of life.

6.  Ensuring that all the providers of care and the patient know the care plan, have input into the care plan, and get regular reports on the progress of the patient according to the care plan.

## Care Plans

*Care plans* are used for DM and case management. The DM care plan is usually a general plan of care that is applicable to a large population with one disease or condition. The care plan for case management is usually individualized for the patient. The following process is an example of how an individual care plan is developed.

1.  Identify the patient who needs a case management care plan. This may be done through the use of claims data, predictive modeling, or other sources of information.

2.  Assign a case manager to the patient.

3.  Identify the diagnosis of the patient, how the case was referred.

4.  Initiate patient assessment. This can be done using proprietary or off-the-shelf programs. The assessment should be for the patient's specific medical condition.

5.  Coordinate with the providers of care after the assessment to determine their input to the assessment and a plan of care.

6.  Develop a care plan, utilizing the inputs from the patient, the provider, and the other identified stakeholders of the patient. This care plan includes patient-identified areas for improvement and motivation to improve, and provider-identified milestones of care that will get the member to the best outcome. Identify processes that will remove nonclinical obstacles that will be barriers to the success of the patient and the care plan.

7.  Communicate the care plan to patient, provider, and other stakeholders under HIPAA requirements and get their sign-off.

8.  Continuously update the care plan and the progress made, changing it as needed with inputs from the patient, the provider, and the stakeholders.

9.  Identify timeline and outcomes for the complete case management care plan.

Having an electronic or Web-based system to produce, to disseminate, and to update the care plan makes it easier to be successful in meeting the case management goals and the objectives for the patient. The care plan for disease management would be very similar to the case management process, except it would be more uniform for the patients identified with the specific disease under the DM program. It should be noted that DM and case management are integrated. Often patients who are identified in DM get rolled into case management because their disease process becomes so severe that they need individual case management to improve. Conversely, patients who are finished with case management get rolled into the DM program because their underlying disease is not cured and the patients continue to need self-improvement strategies.

## Demand Management

*Demand management* includes the activity and interventions specifically designed to improve the appropriateness of members' use of health care resources. It may include member self-management, stepped care programs, other UM processes, and community and stakeholder outreach. Demand management is implemented through the following activities:

1.  Providing health information to the patient through calls, faxes, e-mail, the Web, or other mechanisms.
2.  Offering preventive services that follow evidence-based guidelines.
3.  Providing case management, disease management, and other supportive services to the patient.
4.  Evaluating the health risks of patients and newly-insured patients to identify preventive interventions and self-care capabilities.
5.  Partnering with community resources to promote the use of local and national programs that can improve health and wellness.
6.  Monitoring the utilization of a patient's services to identify the need for intervention such as care coordination.

Demand management is usually an ongoing process for patients with or without specific chronic diseases. It can be layered on top of case management, disease management, and other UM processes. It also can be utilized to help support caregivers for patients who are unable to care for themselves. Because demand management may duplicate some of the services provided in other programs, a process should be implemented so that duplication of processes and interventions do not confuse the patient or use health care resources that can be more appropriately allocated. Demand management may increase the cost of care by helping the patient improve their use of health care interventions. These may include compliance with medications, using health care education classes at local facilities, and following up on preventive services.

There is often confusion between demand management and case management. Demand management is utilized for all of the population in the benefit plan. It may be directed to groups of beneficiaries who need preventive care, chronic care, or other types of self-motivation and improvement. In all of these cases, demand management is a process of communication for a population needing similar or same services. An example is that of demand management programs sent to the parents of children between the ages of 3 months to 6 years to get their required immunizations. In this case, the demand management program is not associated with a disease process, but a preventive clinical intervention. Demand management is also used for populations with chronic disease. An example is to contact all beneficiaries with an established diagnosis of diabetes to get their eye exams on a yearly basis. On the other hand, case management programs target individuals with chronic and/or catastrophic disease. The case management program is not for a population but for that specific patient with an individualized care plan. In the care plan, processes similar to demand management are used to motivate patients to help in their own care. The bottom line is that demand management is for populations of beneficiaries, and case management is for individual beneficiaries.

## Peer Review

*Peer review* is the evaluation of the necessity, quality, cost, and/or utilization of care–service provided by a health care professional–provider. It is performed by health care professionals or providers from the same discipline (or with similar or essentially equal qualifications) who are not in direct economic competition with the health care professional under review. The peer review process compares the health care professional–provider's performance with evidence-based medicine, his/her peers within the same specialty with similar patients, and examines if the health provider's action is within the scope of the medical or insurance benefit of the patient. Peer review regulatory requirements may vary from state to state (e.g., whether the physician conducting review must be in active practice).

Trending and tracking, the accumulation of occurrences or potential occurrences that may warrant review by a peer or a UM committee, should take place during the peer review process. Generally, there is a standard for frequency of similar issues that would trigger a peer review; there also may be a severity of a clinical intervention that would initiate the process. Each health care organization can develop its own indicators, monitors, and benchmarks for peer review.

Peer review is usually protected as confidential information and should not be released outside of the person or body conducting the peer review. The Health Care Quality Improvement Act of 1986 has given peer review an immunity protection, which may vary according to specific state laws.[12]

The following steps may be used in the process of peer review:

1. Identification of an issue or trend needing peer review from an internal or an external source.

2. Request for medical records and additional information so a comprehensive review can take place.

3. Specific dates of information flow to take place from the provider and the reviewer.

4. Review of documentation by appropriate peer.

5. Reviewer identifies a decision using evidence-based medicine, individual patient condition, and other identified criteria.

6. Reviewer decision is sent to UM committee for their input and decision.

7. Decision is sent to provider for response and corrective action plan (if needed).

8. Provider being reviewed is informed of his/her appeal rights.

Peer review is an important part of UM and quality management. It gives clinicians and other providers a fair hearing process that protects their rights and gives them input into the health care system. Peer review also protects patients from potential risks within the health care system.

# Credentialing

*Credentialing* is the process of obtaining, verifying, and assessing information to determine the qualifications of a health care professional to provide services to a patient. The credentialing process examines the training, the education, and the actual experience of the health care professional. This may include data such as the number of times a surgeon has performed a certain procedure and the clinical outcomes for the patients.

Specific criteria for credentialing are well outlined by many organizations. These include the NCQA, Utilization Review Accreditation Commission (URAC), the Joint Commission, and others. Some states may have specific criteria for health care professionals that must be followed.

The following are the general processes involved in credentialing.

*Primary Source Verification*
   Medical School Graduation
   Residency
   Specialty Boards
   State License
   Drug Enforcement Certificate
   History of Professional Liability
   Clinical Privileges
   Malpractice Insurance
   Work History

*Application and Attestation*
   Reason for any Inability to Perform Essential Clinical Functions
   Lack of Present Illegal Drug Use or Chemical Dependency
   History of Loss of License–Felony Convictions
   History of Change in Privileges or Disciplinary Action
   Correctness and Completeness of Application

*Verification*
   National Practitioner Data Bank
   Health Care Integrity and Protection Data Bank
   Licensure Limitations
   Medicare and Medicaid Sanctions

*Initial Site Visit*
   May Be Required for Primary Care Physicians and Some Specialists

## Criteria for Credentialing

When conducted according to these criteria, credentialing is an up-front process that protects patients, health care systems, and physicians from potential quality and utilization issues. Some health care organizations break the credentialing process into two components. The first is the contracting component, which determines whether the physician meets the criteria to have a contract with the health care organization. The second is the actual clinical appropriateness of the physician to have privileges to care for specific types of patients and/or disease processes. For example, all general surgeons may have a contract to provide surgery to a population, but only some of the general surgeons will have privileges to provide thyroid surgery within their contract.

## Physician Profiles

Physician profiles may be one of the most debated issues in UM and health care in general. Physician profiles can be defined as a summary of data and information specific to a physician or practice, compiled electronically from multiple data sources and appropriate methodology. The data is severity adjusted for the group of patients the physician is seeing and is included in the profile. There should also be an adjustment for outliers that could cause the physician profiles to be inaccurate because of the impact of one or two high-cost, high-risk, or other uncontrollable situations. The profile is used to compare utilization, quality, and outcomes of an individual physician or group of physicians with their peers in a similar geographic area, area of practice, and appropriately adjusted population. Further details on profiling are discussed in Chapters 6 and 8.

## Accreditation and Regulatory Oversight of Utilization Management

UM programs are subject to regulatory oversight that ensures that they are not limiting or inappropriately denying the use of health care by patients. The federal government has specific requirements for participation in Medicare that pertain to UM programs by vendors.

Accrediting organizations include, but are not limited to, the Joint Commission, the URAC, the American Association of Ambulatory Health Care (AAAHC), and the NCQA. Each of these organizations has requirements for UM. An example of the major requirements comes from NCQA's 2008 Health Plan Standards and Guidelines and considers the following[13]:

1. A utilization management structure
2. Clinical criteria for UM decisions
3. Communication services
4. Appropriate professionals
5. Timeliness of UM decisions
6. Clinical information
7. Denial notices
8. Policies for appeals
9. Appropriate handling of appeals
10. Evaluation of new technology
11. Satisfaction with the UM process
12. Emergency services
13. Procedures for pharmaceutical management
14. Triage and referral for behavioral health care
15. Delegation of UM

Each of these standards has substandards that must be met. It should be noted that most of the accrediting organizations do not certify the individual UM program as a stand-alone entity but include it as part of an integrated health care organization certification process.

## CASE STUDY ● ● ●

### *The Utilization Process for Elective Surgeries*

How do the processes and methods of UM work on an actual patient and provider? The following is an example of a patient who has been referred for a hip replacement. The patient sees the orthopedic surgeon, who recommends a hip replacement. The request for the hip replacement is communicated to the UM program, and the patient's clinical history is evaluated against the evidence-based criteria. The procedure is approved through prior authorization, and the patient and surgeon arrange for the hip replacement to take place. The patient will be contacted by the UM program to begin the care coordination process. This will include the completion of a needs assessment for postsurgery care to determine whether the patient can go home with therapy or needs placement in a rehabilitation facility for optimal outcome. The patient may also get a health assessment and SF-12 for future determination of the outcome of care, both physiologic and psychological.

The patient discharge planning process begins on the day of hospital admission. The concurrent review nurse certifies that the admission has taken place and, using evidence-based criteria, determines the appropriate length of stay if no complications take place. On a daily basis, the concurrent review nurse stays in contact with the hospital to collect data and information about the patient and the progress of care. The concurrent review nurse also identifies any potential quality issues that could harm or delay the patient's progress. At the time of discharge, a care plan has been identified for the patient and communicated to the surgeon, the patient, and other stakeholders as identified by the patient under HIPAA requirements. If the patient goes home, the concurrent review nurse calls the patient at a set time to make sure the care plan has been initiated and to see if there are any obstacles that may cause the care plan not to be met. During the UM process, there is a physician advisor who is available to evaluate the processes of care and the UM program. The physician can intervene with the surgeon or other health care professional to make sure the patient gets the best outcome.

# Models of Care

Technically, models of care delivery are not unique to the domain of UM. However, because these models have the potential to change the UM practices of providers, patients, payers, and other stakeholders of health care, they will be discussed in this chapter. A few of the prominent models that are being used or advocated for currently are the Chronic Care Model, the Evidence-Based Medicine and Evidence-Based Management Model, and the Patient-Centered Medical Home.

## Chronic Care Model

This model[14] has become a model of care for people with any condition that requires ongoing self-management and interaction with the health care system. The Chronic Care Model can be applied to systems and patients across various chronic illnesses. The systems that use this form of care delivery can range in size from large multihospital health care organizations to single practitioner practices. Research by the MacColl Institute for Healthcare Innovation has shown that the model's outcomes have been healthier patients, more satisfied providers, and cost savings.[15]

The elements of the model include the following.

### Self-Management Support
This model empowers and prepares patients to manage their health and health care and emphasizes patients' central role in managing their health using effective self-management support strategies that include assessment, goal setting, action planning, problem solving, and follow-up.

### Health System
This element aims to create the culture, organization, and mechanisms that promote safe, high-quality care through open encouragement and systematic handling of errors and quality concerns to improve care.

*Delivery System Design*

The model aims to assure the delivery of effective, efficient clinical care and self-management support through defining roles for each health care team member, and through distributing tasks among team members who follow patients on a regular basis. The care delivered should be culturally sensitive and easily understood by the patient.

*Decision Support*

The model promotes clinical care that is consistent with scientific evidence and patient preferences. Patients should receive information about evidence-based guidelines to encourage their participation.

*Clinical Information Systems*

The model aims to organize patient and population data to facilitate efficient and effective care; make sure that the clinicians use timely reminders for patients and themselves; identify relevant subpopulations for proactive care; facilitate individual patient care planning and monitoring; share information with patients and providers to coordinate care; and continuously monitor the performance of the practice team and the care system.

*The Community*

The model aims to mobilize community resources to meet the needs of patients; encourage patients to participate in effective community programs; partner with community organizations to support and to develop interventions that fill gaps in needed care and services; and advocate for policies and implementations that improve patient care.

## Evidence-Based Medicine and Evidence-Based Management Model

Steven Shortell developed this model of care that links evidence-based medicine and evidence-based management.[16] According to the model, the two components necessary to improve the quality of medical care are (1) advances in evidence-based medicine that identify clinical practices leading to better care, including the content of providing care; and (2) the knowledge of how to put evidence-based medicine into routine practice.

The evidence-based medicine and evidence-based management model utilizes many of the same techniques as the Chronic Care Model. These include disease registries, clinical guidelines, reminder systems, patient self-management education, physician feedback reports, and health care teams. The development of the techniques is enhanced by evidence-based management. The evidence-based management uses knowledge from human factors engineering, high-reliability organizations, changes in organizational culture, development of high-performing teams, identification and correction of mistakes, and the continuous asking of and learning from how an organization improves.

## Patient-Centered Medical Home Model

The medical home is another model that has been around for some time and has been modified over the years by several organizations. The most recent iteration is the Patient-Centered Medical Home (P-CMH) as described by the American Academy of Family Practice, American Academy of Pediatrics, American College of Physicians, and American Osteopathic Association.[17] The patient-centered medical home is defined as an approach to providing comprehensive primary care for children, youth, and adults. In this model, primary care is provided in a health care setting that facilitates partnerships between individual patients and their personal physicians and, when appropriate, the patient's family. The following are the joint principles describing the P-CMH.[17]

1. Personal physician. Each patient has a personal physician who provides ongoing, initial, and comprehensive care.

2. Physician-directed medical practice. The personal physician leads the care team responsible for the ongoing care of the patient.

3. Whole person orientation. The personal physician either provides or arranges for all of the patient's health care needs for all stages of life.

4. Care is coordinated and/or integrated. This model aims for integration across all elements of the health care system and the patient's community. Care is facilitated by registries, information technology, information exchanges, and systems to make sure the patient receives all the care indicated in a culturally and linguistically appropriate manner.

5. Quality and safety are hallmarks of the medical home. Practices support the attainment of optimal, patient-centered outcomes through robust sensitive care planning, evidence-based medicine, and clinical decision support tools that guide decision making; physicians accept responsibility for quality improvement and performance measurement; patients participate in decision making and feedback of their care. As much as possible, information technology is utilized to support patient care, performance measurement, patient education, and enhanced communication. In general, practices have a voluntary outside review to demonstrate their ability to provide patient-centered care; patients and families are part of the practice quality improvement activities.

6. Enhanced access. Patients have appropriate access to their health care through open scheduling, expanded hours, and a variety of communication channels.

7. Payment. In this model, reimbursement recognizes the added value provided to patients and supports the development and compensation necessary to put the P-CMH model in place. It recognizes case-mix differences in patient populations, develops methods to share savings from reduced misuse and overuse of the health care system, and rewards continuous improvement.

## Future Trends

Physician reimbursement will likely drive the future of UM. In California, physician practices are returning to partial or full capitation systems. Capitation reimbursement has driven physicians to be more aware of the use of health care resources and the cost of those resources. In some cases capitation has changed the physicians' use of specialists and/or diagnostic providers because the same outcome and quality can be obtained from one specialty group at a more patient-friendly facility and at a more competitive cost.

P4P is also driving changes in the future of UM. Some P4P programs have identified monitors and indicators of utilization such as referrals per thousand, high-cost diagnostic procedures per thousand, admissions to inpatient facilities per thousand, and overall use of health care dollars per patient. These indicators and monitors, when given back to the physicians along with the money attached to the P4P program, can have a significant impact on how physicians practice and influence their use of evidenced-based medicine. With P4P, in several cases, utilization can be decreased without increasing prior authorization and concurrent review processes and resources.

Information technology will likely streamline the processes of UM. Having Web-based capability with instant approval or denial logic embedded in the software will allow the processes to be faster and to help patients receive their clinical interventions in a timely fashion. Information flow will also decrease duplicate testing and consults, because the information will be Web-based and available for viewing by all providers according to the HIPAA guidelines.

We predict that UM will not be able to be a stand-alone process in the future and will have to be combined with quality, patient safety, and patient empowerment to be successful. By combining all three programs, true and long-term value will be added to the health care system.

## References

1. Flexner A. *Medical Education in the United States and Canada, Number Four: A Report to the Carnegie Foundation for the Advancement of Teaching*. New York: Carnegie Foundation for the Advancement of Teaching; 1910.
2. Codman AE. The product of a hospital. *Surg Gynecol Obstet*. 1914;18:491–496.
3. The Joint Commission. The Now and Future Joint Commission. http://www.jointcommission .org/AboutUs/joint_commission_now_future.htm. Accessed October 16, 2008.
4. Martin PP, Deaver DA. Social Security: A program and policy history. *Soc Sec Bull*. 2005;66(1). http://www.ssa.gov/policy/docs/ssb/v66n1/v66n1p1.html. Accessed October 17, 2008.
5. Luce J, Bindman A. A brief history of health care quality assessment and improvement in the United States. *West J Med*. 1994;160(3):264.
6. Reams BD. *The Peer Review Improvement Act of 1982: A Legislative History of Public Law No. 97-248*. Buffalo, NY: William S. Hein Publishing; 1990.
7. American College of Medical Quality. *Core Curriculum for Medical Quality Management*. Sudbury, MA: Jones and Bartlett; 2005:69–94.

8. National Committee for Quality Assurance (NCQA). Quality Improvement Activity Form Instructions. http://www.google.com/search?sourceid=navclient&ie=UTF-8&rlz=1T4ADBS_enUS294US295&q=NCQA%2c+generic+improvement+activity+form. Accessed October 17, 2008.

9. Milliman, Inc. Milliman Care Guidelines. http://www.milliman.com/expertise/healthcare/products-tools/milliman-care-guidelines/index.php. Accessed October 16, 2008.

10. Qualis Health. McKesson releases InterQual Criteria Version 3.0. http://www.qualishealth.org/news/030501-interqual-update.cfm. Accessed October 17, 2008.

11. The Joint Commission. The role of the risk manager in accredited health care organizations [Chapter 1]. In: *Accreditation Issues for Risk Managers*. Oak Brook, IL: Joint Commission Resources; 2004:3.

12. Health Care Quality Improvement Act. The Health Care Quality Improvement Act of 1986. http://www.hcqia.net. Accessed October 17, 2008.

13. National Committee for Quality Assurance (NCQA). Standards and Guidelines for Accreditation, 2008. http://www.ncqa.org/tabid/691/Default.aspx. Accessed October 16, 2008.

14. The Robert Wood Johnson Foundation. Improving Chronic Illness Care. http://www.improvingchroniccare.org. Accessed October 17, 2008.

15. The Center for Health Studies. MacColl Institute for Healthcare Outcomes. http://www.centerforhealthstudies.org/research/maccoll.html. Accessed October 17, 2008.

16. Shortell SM, Rundall TG, Hsu J. Improving patient care by linking evidence-based medicine and evidence-based management. *JAMA*. 2007;298(6):673–676.

17. American Academy of Family Physicians, American Academy of Pediatricians, American College of Physicians, American Osteopathic Association—Patient-Centered Primary Care Collaborative. Joint Principles of the Patient-Centered Medical Home, February 2007. http://www.pcpcc.net/node/14. Accessed October 17, 2008.

## Additional Resources–Further Reading

Agency for Healthcare Research and Quality: http://www.ahrq.gov

DMAA: The Care Continuum Alliance: http://www.dmaa.org

McKesson InterQual Care Planning Criteria: http://www.mckesson.com/en_us/McKesson.com/For+Payors/Public+Sector/InterQual+Criteria+Products/InterQual+Care+Planning+Criteria.html

PA Health Care Cost Containment Council: http://www.phc4.org

Utilization Review Accreditation Commission: http://www.urac.org

# Chapter 8

# External Quality Improvement: Accreditation, Quality Improvement Education, and Certification

*Toni Kfuri, MD, MPH, CMQ, FACOG, and Nancy L. Davis, PhD*

## Executive Summary

The Office of the Actuary projects that by 2016, health care spending in the United States will reach over $4.1 trillion and comprise 19.6% of the gross domestic product.[1] Under pressure from consumers and in response to exigencies of the marketplace, insurers are screening their network of physicians and monitoring hospitals for quality and access. Their findings of inappropriate variation and unexpected deficiency are generating quality improvement projects across the nation.

We define *external quality improvement* as the review of a physician or health care organization's performance by an external or outside body. Some external review systems have a legal statutory basis and could be mandatory, while others are purely voluntary in nature. Their importance lies in the fact that these approaches are undertaken by independent organizations, sometimes acting on behalf of the federal government, state health departments, or their agencies. Some systems are confidential while others are entirely open to public scrutiny. Their ultimate goals are to review, to evaluate, and to rank health care organizations based on explicit standards and measurements; some result in little or no formal actions while others are linked to significant financial or nonfinancial incentives and sanctions.

Demonstrated gaps in the quality and the demand for cost containment, efficiency-driven, and consumer-oriented health care are putting more pressure on health care organizations to remain compliant with the overlapping roles and responsibilities of external review agencies, which are vested with important duties such as accreditation, physician profiling, public reporting, and benchmarking.

Today, most health care organizations have established quality programs in response to certification requirements or in compliance with federal and state legislation. Physician providers must be credentialed and certified on a regular basis by their state licensing boards. Managed care organization and nursing home participation in Medicare or

Medicaid programs requires compliance with standards from state and federal regulatory agencies. State regulations for health plans doing business in a given state vary in their requirements for review or deeming through accreditation. To qualify for reimbursement from the Centers for Medicare and Medicaid Services (CMS), hospitals must be reviewed by CMS or through accreditation by the Joint Commission. Legislative and regulatory mandates, as well as market demands for accreditation by consumer groups and payers and quality improvement efforts by health care providers, become central to the process of external quality improvement.

This chapter presents information on external quality improvement programs and organizations, taking into account their most recent reports and updated changes. These recent changes will have a direct influence on the accreditation and education processes, taking into consideration a more transparent and objectively assessed credentialing mechanism that reflects an evidence-based and patent-centered quality of care.

## Learning Objectives

Upon completion of this chapter, readers should be able to:

- identify the foremost accrediting agencies and outline their roles and responsibilities;

- discuss the concepts of physician profiling, public performance reporting, and benchmarking;

- describe the Healthcare Effectiveness Data and Information Set (HEDIS) and the Baldrige National Quality Program;

- discuss the certification and credentialing processes and their role in quality improvement; and

- understand the role of continuing education in quality improvement.

## History

Beginning in the mid-1990s, American industries and manufacturers started regaining their competitive edge among industrial nations by adopting total quality management (TQM) and "lean manufacturing" to eliminate waste, thus reducing variation and improving efficiency. However, the relative escalating costs of workforce health benefits kept U.S. manufacturers and businesses at a competitive disadvantage in global markets. In 2007, the average premium for family health coverage through an employer was $12,106, of which covered workers paid an average of $3,281. Since 2001, family premiums for employer-sponsored insurance have increased 78%, while wages have gone up 19% and inflation has gone up 17%.

It is true that our health care system is becoming technologically advanced, yet the escalating cost of care far outstrips any perceived societal gains. The market demand for cost control is compounded by the baby boomers effect. Garrett et al. estimated the impact of population aging on medical costs over the next 5 decades in the United States.[2] Specifically, they found that aging will have a greater impact on per capita costs for diseases for which the ratio of costs for older versus younger patients is greater, such as congestive heart failure (CHF), coronary artery disease (CAD), and diabetes.[2] The projected cost change per capita for aging was 48% for CAD and 75% for CHF, compared to a mere 4% change for asthma.[2] Alemayehu et al. also found that nearly one-third of lifetime expenditures are incurred during middle age and nearly half during the senior years.[3] More than one-third of the lifetime expenditures of those who survive to age 85 will accrue in their remaining years.[3]

The Medicare and Medicaid programs were signed into law on July 30, 1965. Since 1965, a number of changes have been made to these programs. In 1982, the Tax Equity and Fiscal Responsibility Act made it easier and more attractive for health maintenance organizations to contract with Medicare and expanded the center's quality oversight efforts through peer review organizations (PROs). PROs scrutinize medical case records and disallow payment to hospitals whenever a physician's care is judged to be unnecessary or inadequate. The name PRO was officially changed to quality improvement organization (QIO) as per the Federal Register on May 24, 2002, in large part to reflect this new emphasis on population-based quality improvement. CMS contracts with QIOs in 3-year cycles, referred to as "scopes of work."[4] Due to escalating expenditures, and in response to the Balanced Budget Act of 1997, CMS is continually developing quality improvement programs in hospitals, physicians' offices, home health agencies, and nursing homes. The QIO Program is a key component of CMS's broad agenda to improve care for Medicare beneficiaries.[4] CMS's quality agenda includes public reporting of quality measures, known as National Quality Initiatives, to help Medicare beneficiaries make informed choices about local health care services. CMS's quality improvement program includes pay-for-performance demonstrations, payment and coverage policies, collaboration with state agencies to administer survey and certification programs for health care providers, and strategic alliances at the national level to create momentum for transformational change at the local level.[4]

Regulatory efforts to manage quality began in the early 20th century and resulted in the founding of the Joint Commission of Accreditation of Hospitals (JCAH) in 1951. Today, this organization is known as the Joint Commission, and it acts as an independent, non-profit organization whose primary purpose—providing external accreditation—has remained largely unchanged to this day. For several decades, the organization (known as the Joint Commission on Accreditation of Healthcare Organizations [JCAHO] until its most-recent name change in January 2007) also has accredited health care organizations and programs. See Chapter 7 for more detail.

Graduate medical education (GME) received public funding and support for the first time with the passage of the Medicare Bill in 1965 (Medicare Part A). Over the next few decades, the medical education community felt the need to coordinate standards of residency programs to improve the quality of education. In 1968, the AMA set an example for quality standards when it established its Physicians Recognition Award, to reward physicians who continued their medical education in order to remain competent in practice. Soon, many state medical boards set requirements for CME credit to maintain licensure. In 1972—under the direction of the American Medical Association (AMA) and with the support of the American Board of Medical Specialties (ABMS), the America Hospital Association (AHA), and medical colleges—the Coordinating Council on Medical Education (CCME) was formed and charged with approving and coordinating medical education. In 1981, the CCME was abolished and replaced by the Accreditation Council for Graduate Medical Education (ACGME), whose function mainly was limited to accreditation of GME. At the same time, the AMA supported the creation of the Accreditation Council for Continuing Medical Education (ACCME) to accredit medical schools, hospitals, and medical specialty societies as providers of AMA-certified continuing medical education (CME).

## Accreditation

### National Committee for Quality Assurance (NCGA)

There are several external agencies, including regulatory ones that assist with medical quality management and accreditation efforts. We present a synopsis of these agencies that, along with QI efforts, assist in leading to safer and more effective health care systems.

NCQA is a private, 501(c)(3) nonprofit organization dedicated to improving health care quality. Since its founding in 1990, NCQA has been a central figure in driving improvement throughout the health care system and in helping to elevate the issue of health care quality to the top of the national agenda.[5] The range of evaluative programs offered by NCQA is broad and includes accreditation, certification, and physician recognition programs. These programs apply to organizations and individuals ranging from health plans—including health maintenance organizations (HMOs) and preferred provider organizations (PPOs)—to physician networks, medical groups, and even individual physicians.

Survey teams of physicians and managed care experts conduct NCQA's accreditation survey process. In addition to an on-site review, NCQA requires submission of (and includes in the accreditation scoring process) data on key clinical and service measures such as mammography screening rates, smoking cessation efforts, and consumer satisfaction (HEDIS). NCQA's annual publication, *State of Health Care Quality Report*, is produced to monitor and report on performance trends over time, to track variations in patterns of care, and to provide recommendations for future quality improvement.[6]

Among the most remarkable achievements influenced by systematic measurement, reporting, and improvement of quality is the increase in the percentage of heart attack patients who were discharged from the hospital on beta-blocker drugs to prevent second, often fatal, heart attacks. When NCQA began measuring this lifesaving treatment in 1996, fewer than 2 in 3 patients were receiving the right care. But in 2006, more than 97% of heart attack patients received beta-blockers, and nearly every plan that reported on its performance had beta-blocker treatment rates of 90% or higher.[6] This single improvement has saved between 4400 and 5600 lives over the last 6 years, and improved the health of tens of thousands of people.[6] This is a prime example of a successful external quality improvement program that, over a 6-year span, is almost uniformly adopted by health care providers. Notably, this measure has been retired from the HEDIS data set and replaced by a measure of persistence of treatment.

## Utilization Review Accreditation Commission (URAC)

In the late 1980s, concerns grew over the lack of uniform standards for utilization review (UR) services. As a result, the URAC was formed and its first mission was to improve the quality and accountability of health care organizations that use UR programs. In later years, URAC's mission expanded to cover a larger range of service functions found in various health care settings, including the accreditation of integrated systems, such as health plans, and smaller organizations offering specialty services. Now, in its 14th year of operation, URAC has over 16 accreditation and certification programs.[7]

URAC is the largest accrediting body for health care, and it accredits many types of health care organizations. URAC has a number of different accreditation programs—some that review the entire organization (e.g., health plan standards) and some that focus on quality within a single functional area in an organization (e.g., case management, credentialing). Any organization that meets the standards, including hospitals, HMOs, PPOs, third-party administrators (TPAs), health care centers, health plans, health networks, and provider groups, can seek accreditation in case and in health utilization management, including workers' compensation, disease management, consumer education and support programs, recently established standards for health Web sites, HIPAA privacy, and security accreditation programs.[7]

Quality improvement is an essential component of an effective health care organization. URAC's accreditation standards require accredited companies to engage in QI programs relevant to their business operations. In addition, health care organizations are often asked by purchasers and regulators to report on the quality of care. URAC's research activities address a number of priority areas for URAC-accredited companies. Research is being conducted in patient safety, medical management as part of disease management or utilization management, PPOs, workers' compensation, and health informatics.[8]

In January 2005, URAC added its Consumer Education and Support (CES) accreditation program to empower consumers in the growing consumer-directed health care sector. The CES accreditation acknowledges the usefulness of Internet-based general information and targeted messaging to help consumers make better health plan and personal behavior choices.[8] In January 2006, URAC revised all of its standards for health care management organizations by creating a stronger focus on patient safety. Organizations seeking URAC accreditation for medical management programs must maintain at least two quality improvement projects.[9] At least one such project must focus on consumers, and one must focus on error reduction and/or patient safety. In October 2007, URAC announced the first group of companies to achieve Pharmacy Benefits and Drug Therapy Management Accreditations, two new designations intended to optimize therapeutic outcomes and reduce medication errors.[7]

## The Joint Commission

The Joint Commission is the national accrediting body for most hospitals and some other types of health care delivery organizations. Hospitals that request a Joint Commission evaluation of their facility are charged a fee. Because accreditation is not automatically renewed, a full accreditation survey is required at least every 3 years. In 2004, the Joint Commission began using a new accreditation process called Shared Visions–New Pathways, which shifts the focus from survey preparation to a continuous improvement of operational systems that directly affect the quality and safety of patient care.[10] This new accreditation process includes an increased emphasis on periodic performance reviews and on the active engagement of physicians and other caregivers, an on-site survey directed by the priority focus process, and an on-site evaluation of compliance with standards relating to patients' care experience. In 2006, the Joint Commission began conducting on-site accreditation surveys and certification reviews on an unannounced basis.

The Joint Commission evaluates and accredits nearly 15,000 health care organizations and programs in the United States.[11] Their services encompass general, critical access, and childrens' hospitals, as well as psychiatric and rehabilitation institutions. The Joint Commission also certifies medical equipment services, hospices, and other home care organizations, as well as nursing homes and long-term care facilities. Lastly, the Joint Commission also surveys office-based surgical centers and other ambulatory providers, including group practices and independent laboratories.

In order to evaluate the safety and the quality of care provided by their accredited health care organizations, each year the Joint Commission establishes National Patient Safety Goals,[12] which have specific requirements for protecting patients. The changes to the 2007 goals were patient-centered and, for 2008, the Board of Commissioners approved new changes in medication and patient safety (Table 8-1).[12]

Laschober et al. found that large Joint Commission-accredited hospitals are giving more consideration to practice guidelines and the internal sharing of quality measure results and are increasing their investment in quality improvement projects, people, and systems in order to increase documentation of care.[13] At the Cleveland Clinic, Michota is bridging the gap between evidence and practice in venous thromboembolism (VTE) prophylaxis by using a quality improvement program, implementing the National Quality Forum–Joint Commission-endorsed standards, and identifying key features of a successful improvement strategy for prevention of VTE.[14] However, Leonardi and colleagues' review of available national hospital comparison Websites, including the Joint

| TABLE 8-1 Recent Changes to National Patient Safety Goals | |
| --- | --- |
| **2007 National Patient Safety Goals** | **2008 National Patient Safety Goals** |
| • The complete list of medications is provided to the patient on discharge from the facility. | • Reduce the likelihood of patient harm associated with the use of anticoagulation therapy. |
| • Encourage patients' active involvement in their own care as a patient safety strategy. | • Improve recognition and responses to changes in a patient's condition. |
| • Define and communicate the means for patients and their families to report concerns about safety and encourage them to do so. | • Measure and assess, and, if appropriate, take action to improve the timeliness of reporting and the timeliness of receipt by the responsible licensed caregiver of critical test results and values. |

*Adapted from:* The Joint Commission. National Patient Safety Goals. http://www.jointcommission.org/PatientSafety/NationalPatientSafetyGoals. Accessed May 31, 2008.

Commission site, showed "suboptimal measure of quality and inconsistent results," which could be partially due to a lack of complete and timely data.[15]

The Joint Commission developed the Sentinel Event policy in support of its mission of health care safety improvement. A *sentinel event* is defined as "an unexpected occurrence involving death or severe physical or psychological injury, or the risk hereof," including unanticipated death or major loss of function unrelated to the patient's condition.[12] Once a sentinel event has occurred, the health entity must perform a detailed system analysis, such as a root-cause analysis, to review the facility's failed performance that led to the accident and to initiate an action plan. The Joint Commission could start its own sentinel event investigation in cases of continuous threat or noncompliance by the health care institution. This quality improvement tool is the basis for the yearly updates and the changes to the Commission's National Patient Safety Goals.[12]

The 2007 medical staff standards of the Joint Commission changed the peer review process by strengthening *focused evaluation* (Medical Staff [MS].4.30), an intense assessment of a practitioner's credentials and current competence, as it applies to new applicants for medical staff positions and to practitioners demonstrating negative performance. The hospital must confirm with primary sources the obligatory current training, knowledge, skills, and abilities of the applying practitioner. It also could involve the evaluation of a practitioner's performance via proctoring by a peer practitioner.[10] *Ongoing evaluation* (MS.4.40) goes beyond the traditional peer review that applies to practitioners who already have been granted privileges, by requesting reliable practice outcome and performance data.[10] These assessments will be done at least every 2 years for all medical staff members who must undergo a practice evaluation for recredentialing and renewed privileges.

## The Leapfrog Group

In November 2000, a number of large employers and public purchasers founded the Leapfrog Group in an attempt to unify the voice of health care purchasers and to engage consumers and clinicians in improving health care. It developed this approach with many of the nation's largest corporations and in partnership with public agencies, such as the CMS, the U.S. Office of Personnel Management, and the Department of Defense. The Leapfrog Group includes more than 160 private- and public-sector purchasers, who together buy benefits for more than 37 million Americans in all 50 states.[16]

The Leapfrog Group's mission is to "trigger giant leaps forward in the safety, quality and affordability of health care."[16] Four hospital quality and safety practices are the focus of Leapfrog's hospital rating program (Table 8-2).

Today, the Leapfrog Group collects hospital data from 1300 hospitals, covering more than 58% of all hospital beds.[16] (Hospital ratings are available on their Website.) Results of a survey released in September 2007 show that just over half (52%) of U.S. hospitals reporting to Leapfrog indicate they have adopted the Leapfrog Never Events policy. Those hospitals pledge to apologize to the patient and/or the family in the event of a rare medical error. They also agree to report the event, perform a root-cause analysis, and waive all costs associated with the harmful event.[16] This is a good example of the influence of an external QI organization on improving the quality and safety of health care services.

## International Organization for Standardization (ISO)

The International Organization for Standardization (ISO) is the world's largest developer and publisher of international standards and comprises a network of the national standards institutes of 155 countries.[17] The vast majority of ISO standards are specific to a particular process or industry; however, ISO 9001 is specific for quality, and yet, is a

---

TABLE 8-2   **Leapfrog's Quality and Safety Practices**

| | |
|---|---|
| CPOE | Enter medication order via computer, linked to prescribing error prevention software. |
| EHR | Evidence-based hospital referral, hospitals with extensive experience, best results. |
| IPS | Staffing ICUs with physicians with special training in critical care medicine. |
| Score | National Quality Forum-Endorsed 30 Safe Practices to reduce risk of harm. |

*Adapted from:* The Leapfrog Group. Fact Sheet. http://www.leapfroggroup.org/about_us/leapfrog-factsheet. Accessed July 28, 2008.

"generic standards management system," meaning that the same standard can be applied to any organization, large or small, in any sector, and to any business, government agency, or health care entity.[17]

ISO 9001:2000, the world's foremost quality management system, provides the actual requirements an organization must comply with. The standard is highly generic and versatile and is applicable to all health care organizations, regardless of their size or subsector. ISO 9001:2000 can lead to improvement in care process, cost reduction, and the potential for efficiency gains.[17] Goals of ISO standards focus on improved product quality and reliability with adherence to health and safety production standards, cost-effectiveness, and reduction of waste. ISO 9001 is a useful framework with which to evaluate and to improve quality and operations within a health care organization.

If a health care provider is certified to ISO 9001, any other survey process for health care quality certifications will be much simpler and less costly regarding both preparation and compliance demonstration. ISO certification helps improve documentation and records, while focusing on patient care, satisfaction, and safety. While ISO is not intended to replace the Joint Commission, URAC, NCQA, or CMS, it does make the compliance demonstration process much easier to manage, less time consuming, and less costly.[17] The international standards that are available for the health care industry are displayed in Table 8-3.

## Profiling

Physician profiling is a process whereby doctors are rated on measures and standards of quality of care and cost efficiency. Such profiling relies on the growing practice of creating electronic medical records. Once kept only on paper, records about patients, doctors, hospitals, pharmacies, and other caregivers are increasingly aggregated in giant digital storehouses, although most profiling is still done using individual health plan databases on physicians. Analysts assess cost efficiency by looking at factors such as how many and what types of exams were conducted. Was magnetic resonance imaging indicated for investigating migraine? Or, was this medication appropriate for that diagnosis? Doctors are then rated against peers in the same community, by type of patient and illness, and against clinical performance guidelines.

| TABLE 8-3 | International Standards Available for Health Care | |
|---|---|---|
| TC 215 | Health Informatics | Health Information/Communication Technology |
| TC 76 | Transfusion | Infusion/Injection Equipment/Containers and Vials |
| TC 150 | Implants | Surgical Implants/Instrumentation/Terminology |
| TC 210 | Quality Management | Medical Devices/Requirements/Guidance |

*Adapted from:* International Organization for Standardization Website. http://www.iso.org/iso/standards_development/technical_committees/list_of_iso_technical_committees.htm. Accessed July 29, 2008.

Some private health plans have tried to control large variations in practice patterns across physicians to hold down spending, either by influencing the patient's choice of doctors or by limiting physicians' resource use. One approach has been to reduce co-payments to lower-cost physicians. Patients also can choose their doctors based on the public ranking of those physicians' utilization patterns and intensity of treatments. Confidential feedback to physicians has been used by managed care organizations to educate doctors, to modify how they practice, and ultimately to lower costs of care. Higher efficiency practices will be rewarded financially and profit from pay-for-performance plans of care.

Per capita and episode profiling approaches may yield particularly useful information when combined. This is illustrated by the Medicare Payment Advisory Commission's (MedPAC) analysis of seemingly contradictory findings.[18] In lower episode costs, physicians could have higher per capita spending; however, because they were more likely to identify patients as having the disease, the outcome was that more episodes were identified. According to the MedPAC analysis, for example, patients in Miami with coronary artery disease presented with, on average, nearly three episodes of the disease, compared with approximately two episodes per patient in Minneapolis. The implication of these findings, according to the analysis, is that physicians in Minneapolis directed a more intensive style of care for patients more likely to need treatment for the disease.[18]

Dumit writes in the September 2007 issue of the *National Health Policy Forum* that CMS is moving forward with plans to engage in profiling slowly at first, with an initial feedback report to physicians.[19] Resistance is anticipated to come from physician providers, while compiling the data and adjusting their profiles. Dumit states that:[19]

> While few would disagree with the notion that providers should be efficient in the delivery of healthcare services, few would agree on what services should be cut out to improve efficiency. Unless a profiling effort adequately accounts for differences across patients and outcomes, it would be criticized as inappropriately targeting particular physicians or high-cost patients.

Dumit adds:[19]

> Unless the data were shown to accurately reflect a physician's practice pattern, they would be discredited as unfair. Each of these methodological issues alone is a high hurdle. Given the Medicare program's ongoing struggles to rein in spending growth and the evidence on inefficient practice, however, efforts to scale these hurdles may reap benefits in the long run. Medicare's involvement will be an important catalyst for refined data tools and methods that could benefit everyone in the healthcare arena.

Risk adjustment remains a difficult hurdle, especially regarding the selection of risk adjustors and statistical approaches affecting physician profiles. In comparing the performance of physician groups on patient satisfaction with asthma care, Huang et al. found that the use of sociodemographic, clinical, and health status variables maximized risk-adjustment model performances.[20] The "selection of risk adjustors had more influence on ranking profiles than choice of statistical strategies."[20] (p.40) Finally, Thomas et al. identified no consistent combination of outlier methodology and episode attribution rule to be superior for identifying cost-inefficient physicians.[21]

## Healthcare Effectiveness Data and Information Set (HEDIS)

HEDIS is a tool used by more than 90% of America's health plans to measure performance on important dimensions of care and service.[5] Point-of-service (POS) plans and HMOs have a long history of reporting quality data; however, a growing number of PPOs are also reporting on the quality of care they deliver in response to NCQA's call, in 2005, to voluntarily report HEDIS data.[5] HEDIS makes the performance data of different health plans available to health care purchasers, allowing them to make objective comparisons and decisions regarding their coverage.

HEDIS measures address a broad range of important health issues, as reported in the 2007 *State of Health Care Quality Report:*[6]

- Use of appropriate medications for people with asthma
- Management for patients with cardiovascular conditions
- Controlling high blood pressure
- Antidepressant medication management
- Breast, cervical, and colorectal cancers
- Comprehensive diabetes care

This latest report revealed a "surge" in quality reporting, especially in PPOs. Those plans that chose to report their data performed well compared to HMOs and POS plans. As reported earlier in this chapter (see section on NCQA), performance with regard to beta-blocker treatment was very good, approaching 90% or higher.[5] The report also mentions the poor performance of private plans participating in Medicare, which demonstrated improvement in only 8 of 21 measures of effectiveness of care.[6] Measures of mental illness treatment have shown little improvement over many years of data, indicating an urgent need for policy assessment of mental health treatment and reimbursement plans.[6]

Included in HEDIS is the Consumer Assessment of Healthcare Providers and Systems (CAHPS) 4.0 survey, which is a tool for gathering and reporting information on consumers' and patients' experiences with health care services. CAHPS measures of consumer experience, as reported in this year's *State of Health Care Quality*, include the following:[5]

- Claims processing
- Getting care quickly

- Getting needed care
- How well doctors communicate
- Rating of health care
- Rating of health plans
- Rating of personal doctors
- Rating of specialists

In 2008, the survey will also report on the health plan experiences of commercial and Medicaid members.[5]

# Baldrige

The Malcolm Baldrige National Quality Improvement Act of 1987 was signed by President Reagan, establishing the program and making quality a national priority. Today, the Baldrige National Quality Program is being modeled in more than 40 states, Europe, and the Far East.[22] The Baldrige Criteria for Performance Excellence are widely used as an assessment and improvement tool.[22] In 1999, categories for education and health care were added to the original three categories of manufacturing, service, and small business. In 2007, a nonprofit category was added. Through 2005, 68 award recipients have been selected across five categories, including five health care organizations.[22]

The Baldrige Health Care Criteria are designed to help organizations use an integrated approach to organizational performance management, resulting in the goals found in Table 8-4. The 2008 cycle reflects more interest coming from the health care industry, with close to 50% of applicants coming from health care organizations.

The Baldrige Criteria are embedded in core values and concepts. They are applicable to high-performing health care organizations that are integrating key performance and operational requirements within a results-oriented framework, creating a basis for action and feedback. Every health care application is examined and scored by consensus on a point value system. Every applicant receives a detailed feedback report based on an independent external assessment conducted by a panel of specially

---

TABLE 8-4   **Health Care Criteria for Performance Excellence Goals**

| | |
|---|---|
| • Improved health care quality | • Delivery of value to patients |
| • Improved organizational sustainability | • Delivery of value to customers |
| • Improved organizational effectiveness | • More effective health care provider |
| • Improved organizational capabilities | • More capable health care provider |
| • Improved organizational learning | • Improved provider learning |

*Adapted from:* Baldrige National Quality Program. 2008 Health Care Criteria for Performance Excellence. http://www.baldrige.nist.gov. Accessed May 31, 2008.

TABLE 8-5    2008 Health Care Criteria for Performance Excellence–Item Listing

| Criteria | Item Listing | Point Values |
|---|---|---|
| 1. Leadership | 1.1 Senior leadership | 70 |
| | 1.2 Governance and social responsibilities | 50 |
| 2. Strategic planning | 2.1 Strategy development | 40 |
| | 2.2 Strategy deployment | 45 |
| 3. Focus on patient, customers, and markets | 3.1 Patient, customer, and market knowledge | 40 |
| | 3.2 Patient relationships and satisfaction | 45 |
| 4. Analysis and knowledge management | 4.1 Measurement and analysis of organizational performance | 45 |
| | 4.2 Management of information technology | 45 |
| 5. Workforce focus* | 5.1 Workforce engagement | 45 |
| | 5.2 Workforce environment | 40 |
| 6. Process management* | 6.1 Work systems design | 35 |
| | 6.2 Work process management and improvement | 50 |
| 7. Results | 7.1 Health care outcomes | 100 |
| | 7.2 Patient-focused outcomes | 70 |
| | 7.3 Financial and market outcomes | 70 |
| | 7.4 Workforce-focused outcomes | 70 |
| | 7.5 Process effectiveness outcomes | 70 |
| | 7.6 Leadership outcomes | 70 |
| | | Total Points: 1000 |

*Categories 5 and 6 have been redesigned.

*Adapted from:* Baldrige National Quality Program. 2008 Health Care Criteria for Performance Excellence. http://www.baldrige.nist.gov. Accessed May 31, 2008.

trained and recognized experts.[22] The 2008 Health Care Criteria and items are displayed in Table 8-5.

The criteria for performance excellence emphasize continuous performance improvement, innovation, and integration of processes and results. The Baldrige Criteria, Lean, and Six Sigma are complementary; many organizations use Baldrige to develop an overall performance map to identify areas that need improvement, then use Six Sigma, Lean, or both to design operations or improve processes within the organization.[22]

The Baldrige process is a voluntary system of external quality improvement. Its health care criteria are built around the delivery of patient-centered care by a strong workforce that has visionary leadership. It also looks toward the future with a focus on results and creating value and improvements in health care processes and outcomes.[22] The recipient of the 2005 Baldrige Award in health care was Bronson Methodist Hospital in Kalamazoo, Michigan, and the 2006 winner was the North Mississippi Medical Center, a nonprofit health care delivery system serving 24 rural counties in northeast Mississippi and northwest Alabama.[22] On November 20, 2007, President Bush and Commerce Secretary Gutierrez announced that five organizations were the recipients of the 2007 Malcolm Baldrige National Quality Award, the nation's highest presidential honor for organizational performance excellence. Two were health care organizations: Mercy Health System in Janesville, Wisconsin, and Sharp Healthcare in San Diego, California.

## CASE STUDY ● ● ●

### *The Baldrige Application*

This case study is adapted from the National Institute of Standards and Technology, Technology Administration, Department of Commerce, Baldrige National Quality Program: Arroyo Fresco Community Health Center Case Study. The full case study is available at: http://www.quality.nist.gov/Arroyo.htm. *Please note:* This is a hypothetical applicant (AF Health System) used for Baldrige training exercises.

**Abbreviations used in the hypothetical case:**

- *AF:* Arroyo Fresco, which in Spanish means "cool, flowing stream."
- *CHCs:* Community Health Centers, which are nonprofit, community-owned organizations like AF that provide primary and preventive services to the underserved and strive to improve access and eliminate health disparities regardless of people's ability to pay.
- *CM:* Clinical microsystem, which is a small group of providers along with their patients, processes, information, and information systems. The elements of a CM are interdependent and share a common purpose.
- *VMV:* Vision, mission, and values.
- *Takt Time:* The pace of production or service delivery needed to meet customer demand.

**(A) Question from the 2006 Health Care Criteria for Performance Excellence Category 4.1**

> **4.1 Measurement, Analysis, and Review of Organizational Performance: How do you measure, analyze, and review organizational performance? (45 pts).**
>
> Describe *how* your organization measures, analyzes, aligns, reviews, and improves its *performance* as a health care provider at all *levels* and in all parts of your organization.
>
> Within your response, include answers to the following questions:
> *a. Performance Measurement*
>     (1) How do you select, collect, align, and integrate data and information for tracking daily operations and for tracking overall organizational *performance*, including

progress relative to *strategic objectives* and *action plans?* What are your *key* organizational *performance measures?* How do you use these data and information to support organizational decision making and *innovation* as a health care provider?

(2) How do you select and ensure the *effective* use of *key* comparative data and information to support operational and strategic decision making and *innovation?*

(3) How do you keep your *performance* measurement system current with *health care service* needs and directions? How do you ensure that your *performance* measurement system is sensitive to rapid or unexpected organizational or external changes?

**(B) Written Response of the Hypothetical Applicant for Category 4.1: AF *Health System***

## *Performance Measurement [Category 4.1a]*

### Select, collect, align, and integrate data [Category 4.1a (1)]:

A key element of AF's measurement, analysis, and review of organizational performance is its automated FOCUS scorecard, which uses a commercially available balanced scorecard software application customized to reflect the key measures needed by AF to track daily operations and overall organizational performance. As part of the Strategic Planning Process, a cross-location team representing all the CMs and functional groups (affectionately referred to as the "Data Docs") reviews the performance data from the prior year against AF's VMV and strategic objectives. Roger Sinclair leads the team, which evaluates each measure for its ability to provide timely information, and he helps the team identify any measures required or recommended by a state or national organization, such as hand-washing and other safety measures required by the Joint Commission. The cross-functional makeup of the Data Docs ensures that the data collected for the functional groups align with the health care services delivered by the CMs, and the team's broad representation also results in innovative approaches to measurement. For example, in 2004, some measures associated with Lean were added to track cycle time in several clinical processes, and Takt Time calculations helped to smooth out appointment scheduling.

The senior leadership team reviews and approves all key organizational performance indicators that will be part of AF's FOCUS scorecard. Each CM team may add a few customized measures to track performance against specific services it provides or to reflect the special needs of its patient groups. However, all CM teams track measures that roll up into system measures, such as performance for congestive heart failure, immunization rates, and preventive health care measures. The figure below lists some of the key organizational performance measures found on the FOCUS scorecard. Although not presented in this application due to space limitations, most measures are drilled down into multiple relevant segments, such as age, ethnicity, gender, location, clinical condition, staff category, and CM team.

AF's FOCUS strategic objectives:

| Strategic Objectives (Figure 2.1-2) | Related Action Plan(s) | Sample Measure(s) | Responsibility* | Figure(s) |
| --- | --- | --- | --- | --- |
| **Financial Performance** | | | | |
| Increase net income by decreasing overall cost-to-serve through reductions in administrative and indirect patient costs. | Improve return on assets in clinical units. | RVUs per net asset value | O, C | 7.3-4 |
| | Improve collection rates. | Collection rates | O | 7.3-2–7.3-3 |
| **Organizational Learning** | | | | |
| Take advantage of available internal and external resources to fill workforce gaps. | Provide current staff the time and resources to expand their skills. Provide online learning opportunities/paid time off for study. | Staff proficiency rates | O, C, M | 7.4-3a, 7.4-4a,b, & 7.4-5 |
| | Actively recruit and train volunteers with targeted skills, especially retired health care professionals in the region. | Volunteer proficiency rates | O, C, M | 7.4-3b |
| | Promote enrollment in development programs in health care professions. | Staff and volunteer enrollment rates | O, C, M | 7.4-5 |
| | Increase the grant funding for training and scholarships. | Grant success rate | O | 7.5-8 |
| **Satisfaction** | | | | |
| Improve satisfaction on staff survey "employer of choice" dimensions. | Address lower-scoring issues identified in the most recent Staff Satisfaction Survey. | Staff satisfaction scores | O, M | 7.4-2a,b, 7.4-6a,b |
| Improve external stakeholders' satisfaction. | Address lower-scoring issues identified in the most recent patient, community, and partner satisfaction surveys. | Satisfaction scores | O, C, M | 7.2—all, 7.4-7 |

*O = Organization level, C = Country level, M = CM level

## Comparative data [Category 4.1a (2)]:

Multiple sources of comparative data are available to AF, including the highly relevant peer comparisons from the state CHC Benchmarking Consortium. In keeping with its VMV, AF selects the best available comparison from any source to challenge itself to the highest known standard of excellence. These values are included on the FOCUS scorecard. On a quarterly basis, the senior leaders and the leadership teams at each clinic use the comparative data to identify gaps in performance and define targets for improvement. If specific actions for improving the performance are not known, a team will be chartered to identify them, using the OASIS Improvement Model. For example, CMs compared their results for breast cancer screening rates, and high-performing teams shared their approaches to scheduling, patient follow-up, and staff motivation with lower-performing teams to improve performance organization-wide.

## Keep performance measurement system current [Category 4.1a (3)]:

The health care industry is dynamic, and AF's measures and data collection methods must quickly adapt to new trends. For example, with the implementation of the electronic health record in 2002, data-gathering techniques were rapidly converted to eliminate the need for manual collection of much of the clinical data for the measurement system. AF works with the State Association of CHCs to reevaluate measures each year to ensure that operational definitions are updated, and senior leaders stay current with emerging trends through their participation in various associations and health care forums.

Since the Data Docs include both clinical and administrative staff, they can evaluate performance across the breadth of FOCUS measures and recommend changes in multiple dimensions. For example, after reviewing its performance for treating CHF, a La Paz family medicine CM asked the Data Docs to add new measures to the FOCUS scorecard in 2005: Left Ventricular Function measurement and ACE inhibitor (ACEI) use under "Clinical," CHF visits under "Utilization," and ACEI cost under "Financial." Results are available for only 9 months (and therefore not reported), but there is evidence of improvement, with only a slight increase in the number of CHF visits and an actual reduction in ACEI cost related to the introduction of a generic drug into the formulary (the result of an OASIS project conducted by administrative and clinical staff).

## (C) Scoring on Category 4.1 and Feedback Report to Applicant: *AF Health System*

Your score in this criteria item for the consensus stage is in the 50–65 percentage range. According to the "Scoring Guidelines," this percentage range represents the following:

- An *effective, systematic approach*—responsive to the *overall requirements* of the item—is evident. (A)
- The *approach* is *well-developed*, although *deployment* may vary in some areas or work units. (D)
- A fact-based, *systematic* evaluation and improvement *process* and some organizational *learning* are in place for improving the efficiency and *effectiveness of key processes*. (L)
- The *approach* is *aligned* with your organizational needs identified in response to the Organizational Profile and other Process Items. (I)

**Strengths:**

- AF utilizes a cross-location team, the Data Docs, to review measures; this helps to ensure that selected measures are aligned and integrated. Data from this team then are used during the annual Strategic Planning Process. In addition, measures are used for tracking daily operations, and the automated FOCUS scorecard tracks overall organizational performance.
- AF uses multiple sources of comparative data, including state CHC benchmarking consortium comparisons that are included on the FOCUS scorecard and reviewed quarterly by senior leaders. These data are utilized to identify performance gaps and define targets for improvement.
- AF works with the State Association of CHCs to reevaluate measures each year to ensure that operational definitions are current. The Data Docs team routinely evaluates and assesses measures. This systematic evaluation process allows senior leaders to keep current with emerging trends.
- Senior leaders, clinic leadership, CMs, functional groups, and staff members review and analyze the FOCUS scorecard. Progress toward goals is quickly assessed through coded stoplight colors and the use of control charts for some measures to provide early indication of adverse trends. The OASIS Improvement Model is used to address statistically significant performance issues.
- The three "highs" (high cost, high risk, and high volume) are used to prioritize opportunities for continuous improvement, with deployment initiated by a CM, functional group, or senior leaders.

**Opportunities for improvement:**

- AF utilizes multiple sources of comparative data to challenge its performance in setting targets for improvement; however, comparative data from community-based private medical/dental/behavioral health providers are not evident. The lack of local community level data may affect AF's ability to assess relative performance and provide input into strategic decisions.
- While the Data Docs team evaluates performance in multiple dimensions to keep AF's performance measurement systems current, it is not evident how the performance measurement system is sensitive to rapid or unexpected organizational or external changes.
- While AF deploys improvement priorities to staff, it is not clear how initiatives are deployed to suppliers, partners, and collaborators. This may affect AF's ability to provide innovative care given its reliance on key suppliers and partners to deliver health care services.

# Public Reporting

Many national and state initiatives are under way to mandate that health care organizations publicly disclose information regarding their providers' outcome results. There is a growing consumer demand for health care information that will enable the individual to make informed choices about their health care services. With the rise of high-deductible health plans, patients are being asked to make many more care and cost decisions. Because complex factors are involved in making good health care choices, consumers need clearly understandable comparative information. Similarly, health insurers want more information about which hospitals offer the best quality and value so that they can include those hospitals in their coverage networks.

Public reporting of health care institutions began with rankings of the best hospitals in the nation, based on mortality rates, medical errors, and possible infection rates. Such efforts have been successful at the state level, as have those at the agency and federal government levels. An important strategy is the public dissemination of timely, relevant, and reliable information on health care quality that can be used effectively by the consumer, health care payers, and hospitals. Advocates for public reporting argue that it will inject competition into the health system. In addition, it could help providers improve by benchmarking their performance against others, encourage private insurers and public programs to reward quality and efficiency, and help patients make informed choices.

Studies of current efforts have found that public reporting can add value, but the reports must be carefully designed. The hospital's response to public reporting has been studied by Laschober and colleagues who reported on a 2005 national telephone survey to senior hospital executives and found that:[13]

> Hospital Compare and other public reports on hospital quality measures have helped to focus hospital leadership attention on quality matters. They also report increased investment in quality improvement (QI) projects and in people and systems to improve documentation of care. Additionally, more consideration is given to best practice guidelines and internal sharing of quality measure results among hospital staff. Large, Joint Commission on Accreditation of Healthcare Organizations (JCAHO)-accredited hospitals appear to be responding to public reporting efforts more consistently than small, non-JCAHO accredited hospitals.

Table 8-6 provides a bird's eye view of the process. More specific state agencies are increasingly reporting state data over the Internet.

A recent report by Colmers on *Public Reporting and Transparency*, published by the Commonwealth Fund, advocates that public reporting adds value but must be designed carefully so that erroneous data is not circulated openly. The report also stresses the importance of collaboration between state and federal agencies, with the help of providers and hospitals, so that public reporting becomes a useful and transparent process.[23]

## Certification, Licensure, Credentialing

There is a growing trend among states' licensing boards to use stricter and more complex licensing statutes. This is a result of a growth in the number of unethical practitioners with fake credentials and/or past criminal records and an increased expectation that the public and the media will be made aware of and protected from such criminals.[24] Many state boards continue to improve their licensing process and are trying to expand their jurisdiction over providers across state lines.

TABLE 8-6 Public Reporting Entities Formats and Their Performance Measures

| Public Reporting Entity | Format | Beneficiary | Performance Measures |
|---|---|---|---|
| CMS[a] | QIO Data<br>APU | Nonpublic<br>Providers | AMI, heart (HF)<br>Pneumonia, surgical care |
| The Joint Commission[b] | ORYX | Hospitals | Outcome measures |
| CalHospital Compare[c] | Report card<br>Hospital rating | Consumer<br>health plans | Patient satisfaction measures<br>Patient experience<br>Specific medical conditions |
| Hospital Quality Alliance[d] | Hospital Compare | Public<br>Hospitals | 22 clinical processes<br>30-day mortality |
| National Quality Forum[e] | Hospitals | Consumer<br>Hospitals | Health care-associated<br>infections (HAI) project |
| Institute for Healthcare Improvement[f] | Medical groups<br>Hospitals rating | Consumer<br>Public | Safety, effectiveness,<br>patient-centeredness, timeliness, efficiency, equity |
| The Leapfrog Group | Survey results | Public<br>Payers | Safety survey<br>Hospital quality |
| Healthgrades[g] | Compare data | Physicians<br>Hospitals | Credentials of physicians<br>Hospital rates |

[a]http://www.qualitynet.org
[b]http://www.qualitycheck.org
[c]http://www.CalHospitalCompare.org
[d]http://www.hospitalqualityalliance.org, http://www.qualityforum.org
[e]http://www.qualityforum.org
[f]http://www.ihi.org/IHI/Topics/LeadingSystemImprovement/Leadership/Literature/PublicReportingofHealthCarePerformancein Minnesota.htm
[g]http://www.healthgrades.com/about-us

*Abbreviations:* AMI, acute myocardial infarction; APU, annual payment update; ORYX, Joint Commission Performance System for Home Care Organizations; QIO, Quality Improvement Organization.

Verification of credentials and past practice takes time. According to the AMA:[24]

All states will require proof of prior education and training and proof of the completion of a rigorous licensure examination approved by the board. Specifically, all physicians must submit proof of successful completion of all three steps of the United States Medical Licensing Examination (USMLE). However, because some medical students and physicians had completed portions of the National Board of Medical Examiners and Federation Licensing Examination (FLEX) sequences before the implementation of USMLE in 1994, certain combinations of examinations may be considered by medical licensing authorities as comparable to the USMLE. The USMLE program recommends that such combinations be accepted for medical licensure only if completed prior to the year 2000.

Some states have more stringent requirements and specify that applying physicians pass the USMLE in one attempt at all steps, while other states are more relaxed and will not impose an attempt limit. Postgraduate training requirements for licensure also vary among states; some require a limit of 1 year, while others require up to 3 years, especially for foreign graduates.

As discussed earlier in this chapter, in 2007 the Joint Commission initiated the focused evaluation (MS.4.30), an intense assessment of a practitioner's credentials and current competence conducted by the health care organization that applies to new applicants for medical staff positions and to practitioners with negative performance. The hospital must confirm with primary sources the obligatory current training, the licensure, the knowledge, the skills, and the abilities of the applying practitioner. It could also involve the evaluation of a practitioner's performance via proctoring by a peer practitioner.[10] The ongoing evaluation (MS.4.40) goes beyond the traditional peer review that applies to practitioners with already granted privileges.

Board certification began in 1917 in this country and was first administered to the ophthalmology specialists. The American Board of Internal Medicine (ABIM) was incorporated in 1936; by 2002, a set of shared guidelines and requirements for certification had been agreed upon by the core group of the 24 member boards of the American Board of Medical Specialties (ABMS).[25] Board certification used to be a voluntary system, reflecting the higher standards of excellence of the individual physician. Hospitals and managed care plans were instrumental in pushing the certification process toward a required "preferred" status. Most boards have established a 10-year duration for certification, with the potential for recertification to maintain board status. The recertification process began to be mandatory after 2002, with an added required evaluation of practice performance.[25] The AMA offers up-to-date information on state licensure, including licensing requirements, fees, license renewal, and continuing medical education requirements.[26]

## Teaching Quality Improvement

### Undergraduate Medical Education

In response to the Institute of Medicine's (IOM) Committee on Healthcare in America reports, *To Err Is Human* released in 1999 and *Crossing the Quality Chasm* in 2001, the Association of American Medical Colleges developed the ongoing Medical School Objectives Project (MSOP).[27,28] The project seeks to address two fundamental questions: (1) What should medical students learn about quality of care issues (learning objectives)? and (2) What kinds of educational experiences would allow students to achieve those learning objectives (educational strategies)?[29]

The MSOP groups learning objectives into three main areas:

- The ability to critically evaluate the knowledge base supporting good patient care
- An understanding of the gap between prevailing practices and best practices, and the steps necessary to close that gap
- Participating in closing the gap between prevailing and best practices

Experience has shown that there is no lack of opportunity to integrate quality into medical education, but what is lacking is integration of quality improvement tools (measurement and intervention) and modeling of best practices by faculty and staff.

Additionally, there needs to be a culture change with regard to defensiveness in examining errors and quality issues. The prevalent climate of medical malpractice fears has resulted in the insulation of students and physicians from public accountability. The IOM reports brought this to light and have led to a systematic study of medical errors and quality in health care. With this new mandate, health care professionals are being trained with a new expectation of self-assessment and continuous quality improvement.

As part of the Institute for Healthcare Improvement's (IHI) work to incorporate the teaching of quality improvement into health professional education curricula, eight knowledge domains were identified as essential core content that all health profession students should learn as a part of their training.[30] These are described in Table 8-7.

Assessment of competency in medical education is crucial for quality improvement. Effective assessment tools and faculty development are necessary to ensure that only those students and trainees who are competent advance to the next level of training and, ultimately, to practice. Use of case studies, simulators, and observations in practice will ensure that learners can apply the new knowledge they acquire.

A study conducted by Gould et al. used second-year medical students in community-based primary care practices to collect baseline data for diabetes care, to implement a results-specific intervention, and to reassess quality indicators 6 months later.[31] They found that documentation of specific indicators increased, along with actual improvement of clinical measures. Thus, medical students can be a resource to improve patient care by participating in QI projects in clinical practice.[31]

## Graduate Medical Education

The Accreditation Council for Graduate Medical Education (ACGME) adopted general competencies in 1999 that incorporate the knowledge and recognition of quality of care issues. Implementation of the ACGME's core competencies is being promulgated through the ACGME's *Outcome Project*.[32] The core competencies were later adopted by the ABMS as content for lifelong clinical practice.[33] The six general competency areas are as follows:

- *Patient care.* Provide patient care that is compassionate, appropriate, and effective for the treatment of health problems and the promotion of health.
- *Medical knowledge.* Demonstrate knowledge about established and evolving biomedical, clinical, and cognate (e.g., epidemiological, social-behavioral) sciences and the application of this knowledge to patient care.

## TABLE 8-7  Quality Improvement Knowledge Domains for Health Professions Education

1. *Health care as a process, system.* The interdependent people (e.g., patients, families, eligible populations, caregivers), procedures, activities, and technologies of health care giving that come together to meet the need(s) of individuals and communities.

2. *Variation and measurement.* The use of measurement to understand the variation across and within systems to improve the design and redesign of health care.

3. *Customer–beneficiary knowledge.* Identification of the person, persons, or groups of persons for whom health care is provided or may be provided in the future; an understanding of their needs and preferences and of the relationship of health care to those needs and preferences.

4. *Leading, following, and making changes in health care.* The methods and skills for designing and testing change in complex organizational caregiving arrangements, including the general and strategic management of people and the health care work they do in organizations.

5. *Collaboration.* The knowledge, methods, and skills needed to work effectively in groups, to understand and value the perspectives and responsibilities of others, and the capacity to foster the same in others, including an understanding of the implications of such work.

6. *Social context and accountability.* An understanding of the social contexts (i.e., local, regional, national, global) of health caregiving and the way that expectations arising from them are made explicit. This specifically includes an understanding of the financial impact and costs of health care.

7. *Developing new locally useful knowledge.* The recognition of the need for new knowledge in personal daily health professional practice and the skill to develop new knowledge through empiric testing.

8. *Professional subject matter.* The health professional knowledge appropriate for a specific discipline and the ability to apply and connect it to all of the above.

*Source:* Institute of Healthcare Improvement. Eight Knowledge Domains for Health Professional Students. http://www.ihi.org/IHI/Topics/HealthProfessionsEducation/EducationGeneral/EmergingContent/Eight KnowledgeDomainsforHealthProfessionalStudents.htm. Accessed July 29, 2008.

- *Practice-based learning and improvement.* Demonstrate the ability to investigate and to evaluate patient care practices, to appraise and assimilate scientific evidence, and to improve patient care practices.

- *Professionalism.* Demonstrate a commitment to carrying out professional responsibilities, to adhering to ethical principles, and to showing sensitivity to a diverse patient population.

- *Interpersonal and communication skills.* Demonstrate interpersonal and communication skills that result in effective information exchange and teaming with patients, patients' families, and professional associates.

- *Systems-based practice.* Demonstrate an awareness of and a responsiveness to the larger context and system of health care and the ability to effectively call on system resources to provide care that is of optimal value.

While ACGME has linked accreditation of graduate medical education programs to demonstrations that residents in training are proficient in the core competencies, there is variability between programs and questions regarding the effectiveness of various teaching methods. This is particularly true of the practice-based learning and improvement and systems-based practice competencies, where quality improvement concepts are most important. A systematic review of the effectiveness of teaching quality improvement to clinicians, conducted in 2007, produced evidence of this variability.[34] Teaching methods included didactic and experiential learning and, while most evaluated learning, few used validated assessment instruments. Assessments of attitudes showed mixed results, and only 8 of 28 studies of clinical outcomes reported beneficial effects. Clearly, more study is needed to ascertain how best to teach the concepts of quality improvement *and* to actually improve clinical outcomes.

Ogrinc et al. developed a framework for teaching medical students and residents systems-based practice and practice-based learning and improvement based on a review of the literature.[35] Training, educational objectives, and methodology recommendations were made depending on the learners' skill levels. For example, students at the novice level might develop an understanding of systems-based practice, measure a process, and try a test of change (e.g., Plan, Do, Study, Act [PDSA] cycle) on a system that is familiar to them. An early resident, with mentoring by faculty, might conduct an assessment of his or her own patients' needs and engage other members of the health care team to implement an intervention for improvement. An advanced resident might build on his or her changes to practice, remeasuring and modifying as needed.

For novice learners, intensive, experiential, interdisciplinary training can facilitate improvements in patient care. Varkey et al. found their interdisciplinary QI curriculum created an opportunity for learners in varying disciplines to learn from each others' successes and failures, to share resources, to develop an understanding of the health system, and to stimulate future professional interactions.[36] The learner team successfully completed a QI project in outpatient medication reconciliation as a part of the curriculum.

## Continuing Medical Education

The melding of quality improvement and continuing medical education (CME) has been discussed for decades but did not become a reality until the introduction of maintenance of certification (MOC) in 2000. It was then that the ABMS determined that board certification of physicians should do more to ensure the continuous competence of physicians. At that time, most certifying boards required a written exam every 6 to 10 years, depending on specialty, to maintain certified status. Some boards required no recertification. Based on the core competencies developed by ACGME and adopted by ABMS, the new requirements for ongoing MOC have four components: Part I, Licensure and Professional Standing, requires a valid, unrestricted medical license; Part II, Lifelong Learning and Self-Assessment, requires educational and self-assessment activities determined by each specialty board; Part III, Cognitive Expertise, requires demonstration of specialty-specific knowledge and skills (proctored exam); and Part IV, Practice Performance Assessment, requires demonstration of the use of best evidence and practices compared to peers and national benchmarks.[33] It is this fourth component that truly calls for the integration of quality improvement and CME.

Certifying boards and the corresponding medical specialty societies have developed modules to fulfill MOC Part IV. Generally, these have been modeled after the PDSA cycle for improvement.[37] In these modules, physicians are asked to perform an assessment of their current practice, which might include a survey or chart abstraction. The results of the assessment are compared with peers and national benchmarks. Next, physicians are directed to interventions for improvement, which may include education or systems-based process interventions. Sometime after implementation of the intervention(s), usually 6 months, the physician is asked to reassess their practice and then compare results to peers and national benchmarks. Once the module is complete, the board-certified physician is credited with completion of MOC, Part IV. Figure 8-1 depicts the

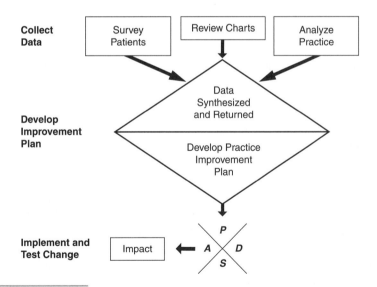

**Figure 8-1**   Diagram on MOC Model: Functional Anatomy of a PIM

*Source:* Holboe ES, Meehan TP, Lynn L, Doyle P, et al. Promoting physicians' self-assessment and quality improvement: The ABIM Diabetes Practice Improvement Module. *J Contin Educ Health Prof.* 2006;26(2):109–119.

process for a Practice Improvement Module (PIM) as required for MOC, Part IV by the American Board of Internal Medicine.[38]

In addition to meeting requirements for MOC, physicians can now receive CME credit for participating in performance improvement activities. In 2005, the AMA, the American Academy of Family Physicians, and the American Osteopathic Association agreed to criteria for awarding CME credit for such activities. Physicians cannot self-report performance improvement CME activities, but must work with an approved CME provider that awards the credit. In order to give added value to performance improvement CME activities, the credit scheme allows participants to receive five credits for each stage of the project: Stage A, practice assessment; Stage B, intervention(s); and Stage C, remeasurement and reflection on new knowledge and practice. When all three stages are complete, the physician is rewarded with five additional credits for a total of 20. This was the first movement away from time as the metric for CME credit. Credit for performance improvement CME is not based on the time the physician spent, but the relative value of the activity. Twenty credits are almost half of the annual CME credit necessary for most physicians for licensure, board certification, and other CME credit requirements.

In 2007, the Accreditation Council on Continuing Medical Education (ACCME) set forth new criteria for accreditation to give incentive to CME providers to integrate quality and performance improvement, collaboration, and higher levels of outcomes measures into their programs.[39] These new criteria came in response to criticism that traditional CME is not effective in improving physician performance and, ultimately, patient care. CME is a $2 billion-plus industry in the United States, over half of which is funded by the pharmaceutical industry.[40] Critics maintain that CME is influenced by that funding and that more emphasis must be placed on evidence-based needs assessment and filling performance gaps in clinical practice. Integrating quality improvement methods and data with educational activities better serves the needs of physicians, the health care system, and the patients they serve.

There are several barriers to integration of CME and quality improvement (QI). QI and CME schools or departments are usually in different areas of organization. This is true in hospitals, medical schools, and other health care organizations. Quality improvement is often viewed as a nursing-oriented function while CME is considered physician oriented. While much rhetoric is devoted to the team approach, it is often difficult to implement. The CME office often is not aware that data is being collected or of the results. Quality management areas see CME as an externally driven and funded activity that is not continuous in nature and that has no overarching, long-term goal that fits into the organization's long-term goals for patient care. Second, education often is not the solution for improving performance. Lapses may not be an issue of "knowing better" but of "doing better." Other systems-based processes or barriers frequently affect practice. Third, many areas of medicine have no evidence-based performance measures. There are no quality data available in many areas where education is needed. CME developers cannot depend on the quality agenda alone to direct their programs. Finally, external funding is crucial to CME units. They often are expected to be at least self-sustaining and preferably profit centers for the organization, and that has led to a dependence on external funding, largely from the pharmaceutical industry, to sustain CME. Organizations fund quality management with the assumption that increased quality will decrease overhead.

How, then, can quality improvement and CME best be integrated? Communication is the key. Staff in the two areas should communicate regularly on a strategic as well as an operational level. Quality improvement priorities of the organization should be a part of the CME program, and individual quality projects should always consider CME as part of the improvement intervention. CME planners should always consider quality data as well as quality improvement processes and tools as part of the educational activity.

Performance data can serve as a needs assessment to identify gaps in knowledge and skills. It can also be used as outcomes data to show if education has an impact on improving physician performance and health care outcomes. Staff who are cross-trained in education and quality can serve both purposes well. Increasing awareness in both disciplines will ensure better utilization and improve effectiveness in both areas.

## Future Trends

As consumers and payers become increasingly interested in performance data, evidence of quality care, continuous pursuit of cost-containment, and efficient strategies to deliver adequate services, external quality improvement will be at the forefront. This will allow accrediting agencies to tighten their processes for more compliance and allow the federal government and payers to demand more accountability for quality and efficient pay-for-performance.

We also believe that teaching quality improvement across the continuum of medical education will become increasingly important. More formal teaching of quality improvement concepts will be introduced to the curriculum and students will be exposed to quality patient safety techniques in the clinical setting. Participation in quality programs, pay-for-performance, and continuing professional development will become a routine part of the physician's professional life.

## References

1. Poisal JA, Truffer C, Smith S, et al. Health spending projections through 2016: Modest changes obscure Part D's impact. *Health Aff.* 2007;26: 242–253.
2. Garrett N, Martini EM. The boomers are coming: A total cost of care model of the impact of population aging on the cost of chronic conditions in the United States. *Dis Manag.* 2007;10:51–60.
3. Alemayehu B, Warner KE. The lifetime distribution of health care costs. *Health Serv Res.* 2004;39:627–642.
4. Centers for Medicare and Medicaid Services, U.S. Department of Health and Human Services. Quality Improvement Organizations: An Overview. http://www.cms.hhs.gov/Quality ImprovementOrgs. Accessed July 29, 2008.

5. National Committee for Quality Assurance. About NCQA. http://www.ncqa.org/tabid/675/Default.aspx. Accessed July 29, 2008.
6. National Committee for Quality Assurance. The State of Health Care Quality Report 2007. http://www.ncqa.org/Portals/0/Publications/Resource%20Library/SOHC/SOHC_07.pdf. Accessed June 3, 2008.
7. Utilization Review Accreditation Commission Website. http://www.urac.org. Accessed June 3, 2008.
8. Utilization Review Accreditation Commission. URAC Research and Grants. http://www.urac.org/research. Accessed June 3, 2008.
9. Utilization Review Accreditation Commission. URAC Consumer Safety Standards. http://www.urac.org/resources/consumerSafety.aspx. Accessed June 3, 2008.
10. The Joint Commission. Fact Sheet. http://www.jointcommission.org/AboutUs/Fact_Sheets/scoring_qa.htm. Accessed July 29, 2008.
11. The Joint Commission. About Us. http://www.jointcommission.org/AboutUs. Accessed July 29, 2008.
12. The Joint Commission. National Patient Safety Goals. http://www.jointcommission.org/PatientSafety/NationalPatientSafetyGoals/08_hap_npsgs.htm. Accessed May 31, 2008.
13. Laschober M, Maxfield M, Felt-Lisk S, Miranda DJ. Hospital response to public reporting of quality indicators. *Health Care Financ Rev.* 2007;28:61–76.
14. Michota FA. Bridging the gap between evidence and practice in venous thromboembolism prophylaxis: The quality improvement process. *J Gen Intern Med.* 2007;22(12):1762–1770 .
15. Leonardi MJ, McGory ML, Ko CY. Publicly available hospital comparison web sites: Determination of useful, valid, and appropriate information for comparing surgical quality. *Arch Surg.* 2007;142:863–868; discussion 868–986.
16. The Leapfrog Group. Fact Sheet. http://www.leapfroggroup.org/about_us/leapfrog-factsheet. Accessed July 28, 2008.
17. International Organization for Standardization Website. http://www.iso.org/iso/home.htm. Accessed July 29, 2008.
18. Medicare Payment Advisory Commission (MedPAC). Report to the Congress: Assessing alternatives to the sustainable growth rate system. March 2007;164–166. http://www.medpac.gov/documents/Mar07_SGR_mandated_report.pdf. Accessed June 3, 2008.
19. Dummit LA. Physician profiling: Can Medicare paint an accurate picture? *National Health Policy Forum Issue Brief.* 2007;825:1–11.
20. Huang IC, Frangakis C, Dominici F, et al. Application of a propensity score approach for risk adjustment in profiling multiple physician groups on asthma care. *Health Serv Res.* 2005, 40:253–278.
21. Thomas JW, Ward K. Economic profiling of physician specialists: Use of outlier treatment and episode attribution rules. *Inquiry.* 2006;43:271–282.
22. Baldrige National Quality Program. 2008 Health Care Criteria for Performance Excellence. http://www.baldrige.nist.gov. Accessed May 31, 2008.
23. Colmers J. Public Reporting and Transparency. January 2007. Report prepared for the Commonwealth Fun/Alliance for Health Reform. 2007 Bipartisan Congressional Health Policy Conference. http://www.commonwealthfund.org/publications/publications_show.htm?doc_id=449503. Accessed July 29, 2008.
24. American Medical Association. Getting a License: The Basics. http://www.ama-assn.org/ama/pub/category/2644.html. Accessed July 29, 2008.

25. Cassel C, Holmboe ES. Professional standards in the USA: Overview and new developments. *Clin Med.* 2006;6:363–367.

26. American Medical Association. Medical Licensure. http://www.ama-assn.org/ama/pub/category/2543.html. Accessed July 29, 2008.

27. Institute of Medicine. *To Err Is Human: Building a Better Health System.* Washington, DC: National Academies Press; 1999.

28. Institute of Medicine. *Crossing the Quality Chasm.* Washington, DC: National Academies Press; 2000.

29. Association of American Medical Colleges. *Contemporary Issues in Medicine: Quality of Care. Report II: Medical School Objectives Project.* Washington, DC: Author; August 2001.

30. Institute of Healthcare Improvement. Eight Knowledge Domains for Health Professional Students. http://www.ihi.org/IHI/Topics/HealthProfessionsEducation/EducationGeneral/EmergingContent/EightKnowledgeDomainsforHealthProfessionalStudents.htm. Accessed July 29, 2008.

31. Gould BE, Grey MR, Huntington CG, et al. Improving patient care outcomes by teaching quality improvement to medical students in community-based practices. *Acad Med.* 2002;77(10):1011–1018.

32. American College of Graduate Medical Education (ACGME). Educating Physicians for the 21st Century: The Outcome Project. http://www.acgme.org/outcome/e-learn/introduction/index.html. Accessed August 1, 2008.

33. American Board of Medical Specialties. Maintenance of Certification Competencies and Criteria 2000. http://www.abms.org/Maintenance_of_Certification/ABMS_MOC.aspx. Accessed September 1, 2007.

34. Boonyasai RT, Windish DM, Chakraborti C, et al. Effectiveness of teaching quality improvement to clinicians. *JAMA.* 2007;298(9):1023–1037.

35. Ogrinc G, Headrick LA, Mutha S, et al. A framework for teaching medical students and residents about practice-based learning and improvement, synthesized from a literature review. *Acad Med.* 2003;78(7):748–756.

36. Varkey P, Reller MK, Smith A, et al. An experiential interdisciplinary quality improvement education initiative. *Am J Med Qual.* 2006;21(5):317–322.

37. Watson M. *The Deming Management Method.* New York: Dodd, Mead; 1986.

38. Holmboe ES, Meehan TP, Lynn L, et al. Promoting physicians' self-assessment and quality improvement: The ABIM Diabetes Practice Improvement Module. *JCEHP.* 2006;26(2):109–119.

39. American College of Continuing Medical Education (ACCME). CME as a Bridge to Quality: Updated Accreditation Criteria. http://www.accme.org/dir_docs/doc_upload/b03aa5cc-b017-4395-a41f-8d5d89ac31ca_uploaddocument.pdf. Accessed July 29, 2008.

40. ACCME. Annual Report Data 2006. http://www.accme.org/dir_docs/doc_upload/f51ed7d8-e3b4-479a-a9d8-57b6efedc27a_uploaddocument.pdf. Accessed July 29, 2008.

## Additional Resources–Further Reading

Accreditation Council for Continuing Medical Education (ACCME). Updated Criteria for Accreditation: http://www.accme.org

American Academy of Family Physicians. Activities Eligible for Prescribed Credit: http://www.aafp.org/online/en/home/cme/selfstudy/metric.html

American Board of Medical Specialties. Maintenance of Certification Competencies and Criteria: http://www.abms.org/Maintenance_of_Certification/ABMS_MOC.aspx

American Medical Association Physicians Recognition Award: http://www.ama-assn.org/ama1/pub/upload/mm/455/pra2006.pdf

Baldrige National Quality Program. Criteria for Performance Excellence: http://www.baldrige.nist.gov

Joint Commission: http://www.jointcommission.org

Mazmanian PE. Advancing the body of knowledge: Evidence and study design for quality improvement. In Davis D, Barnes BE, Fox R, eds. *The Continuing Professional Development of Physicians: From Research to Practice.* Chicago: AMA Press; 2003.

National Committee for Quality Assurance (NCQA): http://www.NCQA.org

Utilization Review Accreditation Commission (URAC): http://www.urac.org

# Chapter 9

# Interfaces Between Quality Improvement, Law, and Medical Ethics

*Jeffrey M. Zale, MD, MPH, CMQ, and Mano S. Selvan, PhD*

## Executive Summary

A solid legal and ethical footing provides the framework and benchmarks for credible, persuasive, accountable quality management activities. Medical quality management should reflect prevailing societal preferences, establishing a balance between the interests of patients, practitioners, institutional providers, health plans, regulatory agencies, and the general public. Legal and ethical standards help to ensure that these preferences are honored and bring clarity and accountability to the process. The quality of care delivered in a facility or health plan is directly influenced by the organization's QI activities, including provider credentialing, risk management, physician and staff oversight, and compliance with the requirements of accreditation and certifying organizations.

As medicine becomes increasingly complex, the legal system is less likely to encompass every aspect. The concepts and tools of clinical ethics and medical quality management processes can be of value in resolving situations that are not well defined in the law or where legal opinion is unclear. Medical ethics helps to improve the quality of patient care by providing a framework to address issues and dilemmas that arise in clinical practice. Patients, families, and health professionals often face difficult decisions with respect to patient care, especially when the right thing to do is not clear, or when uncertainty exists about what is best for a patient. Clinical ethics informs health care decision-making by weighing benefits and risks based on moral values, religious beliefs, or professional duties and guidelines. In a setting with limits on resources, and when health care benefits are restricted or limited, medical quality management decision-making must be done in a transparent and ethical manner.

The purpose of this chapter is to provide a working knowledge of legal and ethical issues related to clinical quality, to provide a context to better understand some of the current challenges, and to provide benchmarks in medical quality management (MQM).

## Learning Objectives

Upon completion of this chapter, readers should be able to:

- identify the basic concepts related to legal and ethical issues in health care;

- discuss the impact of government and court decisions on the practice of medical quality management;

- explain the impact of federal and state laws on health care provision;

- discuss peer review protections and the creation of the National Practitioner Data Bank;

- identify pertinent issues related to HIPAA;

- discuss legal and ethical issues related to medical errors and transparency;

- explain the effects of malpractice, antitrust legislation, and risk management on health care practice;

- present the basic framework for alternatives to litigation; and

- discuss the basic concepts of institutional review boards (IRB) and current controversies in QI.

# History

One of the first documented legal codes was based on Sumerian and Akkadian laws.[1] It was compiled by Hammurabi, who ruled Babylonia between 1795 and 1750 BC.[2] The Code of Hammurabi contains a number of regulations related to what physician actions are permissible, physician payment rates, and reimbursement of the patient for damages as the result of an operation. Under this code, physicians were judged based on quality and outcomes—an ancient pay-for-performance initiative. As societies became more regulated, the legal profession and government increased their oversight, proscribing and prescribing certain actions and activities.

Ethical codes and principles can be found in writings from ancient civilizations in Greece and India. For example, Hippocrates' writings (5th century BC) contain physicians' principles and patients' rights,[3] and Susruta, a renowned Indian surgeon (6th century BC), documented that he required his students to use fruits, vegetables, and artificial models of the human body for surgery training.[4] The basic concepts found in ethical and legal documents evolved in parallel with the development of modern health care. They are embodied in the administrative and financial activities that support the delivery of care, and they are published and disseminated by medical associations.

Peer review, a pivotal element of health care evaluation and oversight, has been fundamental to hospital practice for over a century. When Medicare was signed into law, further peer review requirements were mandated in the form of quality assurance and utilization review activities.[5] The current legal and ethical framework for medical quality management should reflect societal preferences on how to balance the interests of patients, practitioners, institutional providers, health plans, regulatory agencies, and the general public. Legal and ethical standards help to ensure that these preferences are honored.

## Role of Government

The government uses laws and regulations to codify actions it believes to be appropriate in specific circumstances for the protection of the population. These laws and regulations aim to decrease unnecessary variation and complexity.

Federal law preempts state laws in most cases.[5] For example, ERISA (the Employee Retirement Income Security Act of 1974, PL 93-406) establishes minimum standards for pension and other health insurance plans provided by private employers. The act supports private industry by regulating and protecting the interests of employee benefit plan participants and their beneficiaries, by establishing rules of conduct for plan fiduciaries, and by simplifying the creation of multistate or national benefit plans. Because it preempts state law, ERISA permits private companies to offer health plans and benefits nationwide without running afoul of state insurance regulations. In civil lawsuits, ERISA forbids financial awards to beneficiaries for pain and suffering and punitive damages for gross negligence in the mismanagement of the health care plans. This legislation and its impact on certain litigation is at the core of an ongoing debate between state and federal regulations pertaining to the degree of protection and accountability of the fiduciary and the right of the beneficiary to be compensated as a result of harm.

The government supports medical quality professionals through regulations and by providing governmental and government-sponsored organizations such as the Agency for Healthcare Research and Quality (AHRQ), which fosters and facilitates evidenced-based medicine (EBM) and guideline development, and Institute of Medicine (IOM). The IOM, chartered in 1970 as a component of the National Academies of Science, created landmark reports on medical errors, patient safety, and quality improvement[6,7] that spurred the development of national initiatives to improve the quality of health care delivery. In its 2001 report, *Crossing the Quality Chasm*, the IOM challenged health care organizations to take an active role in improving care by focusing on six major areas: safety, timeliness, effectiveness, efficacy, equity, and patient-centered approach.[7] U.S. health care organizations responded by implementing QI activities to make medical care safer for patients.

## Rules, Regulations, Laws, and Acts

The government regulates the practice and delivery of health care through statutes, regulations, rules, and acts. States regulate health care institutions and other health care issues through "public powers," which require that actions be taken to maintain and improve public health and to provide for the safety and welfare of the population of the state. Because both the states and the federal government finance health care services, both can regulate health care provision by defining what care, services, durable medical equipment, and medications are covered under their insurance programs. For example, a participating hospital provider in the Medicare program must agree to physician credentialing, quality-related activities, and other requirements.

Federal health law usually begins as a bill that must be approved by both houses of Congress. As a rule, the laws created in this manner are stated as broad concepts. The details (i.e., rules and regulations) are generally written by the agencies that will administer the laws. In the case of significant rules or regulations—such as the Health Insurance Portability and Accountability Act (HIPAA) or changes to the Medicare reimbursement system—a proposal or draft is published in the Federal Register with a period of time for comments. Responses to the proposal from legislators and the public may result in significant changes. Once the final regulation–rule or act is published, it has the full weight of law.

## Regulation and Public Laws to Ensure Quality

Some laws require quality assurance (QA) activities in addition to QI activities. QA activities focus on compliance with accepted standards or guidelines. In contrast, QI activities focus on measures, processes, and outcomes in an ongoing, iterative course of action to actively improve results.

State-mandated facility inspections and professional licensure constitute the "ground floor" level of quality (i.e., minimum requirements to practice medicine or to provide care in a facility). While licensure is important, it does not ensure high-quality health care.

Some public interest groups, such as Public Citizen, have attempted to use licensure and public sanctions as a measure of the effectiveness of a State Board of Medicine's ability to protect the population. One such method is calculating the proportion of disciplinary actions taken against physicians versus the number of licensed physicians in the state. Such a ratio is potentially misleading as it may include licensed physicians who are not in active practice or are solely involved in research, or do not reside or practice in multiple states where they may be licensed.

States are responsible for a substantial amount of oversight, including licensure, oversight of inpatient facilities and health care professionals, and regulation of non-ERISA managed care and other insurance products. The federal government has a significant impact through the Medicare (federally sponsored) and Medicaid (jointly funded, federal and state sponsored) programs, which affect a high percentage of the population in most states.

States have looked to nationally recognized accreditors, such as the Joint Commission, NCQA, and URAC, as sources for standards. Collecting and reporting NCQA's HEDIS data is a requirement for many state agencies that oversee Medicaid managed care.

Health and safety standards provide a foundation for improving quality and for protecting the health and safety of beneficiaries as inpatients. Governmental oversight and evaluation of the Joint Commission accreditation process is ongoing as evidenced by the GAO-04-850 study. In its Report to Congressional Requesters, *Centers for Medicare and Medicaid Services Needs Additional Authority to Adequately Oversee Patient Safety in Hospitals,* the Government Accountability Office reported that the Joint Commission's pre-2004 hospital accreditation process did not identify a number of the hospitals' deficiencies in Medicare requirements noted by state survey. Suggestions were made to CMS to modify the oversight process.

Many hospitals delegate Medicare oversight to an accrediting agency. The Joint Commission is a private, not-for-profit organization that accredits most of the hospitals that participate in Medicare. Hospitals accredited by the Joint Commission are considered to be in compliance with the requirements for Medicare participation. Under the Medicare statute, Joint Commission-accredited hospitals are considered "deemed" as if they had met requirements for Medicare certification (42 USC §1395x [e] and §1395bb).

As a volume purchaser of health care, CMS affects how care is delivered to seniors and the disabled. It also has a significant impact on commercial insurance carriers and Medicaid. CMS's reimbursement and coverage rules affect a large percentage of hospitalized and ambulatory patients. Changes in Medicare coverage make it necessary for hospitals to modify policies, procedures, staff education, and ongoing oversight for compliance by clinical staff, hospital administrators, and hospital compliance officers.

The Deficit Reduction Act of 2005 directed Health and Human Services (HHS) to identify a number of preventable inpatient complications, the occurrence of which would no longer be reimbursed by Medicare. This new rule, mandated under Section 5001(c) of Public Law 109-171, was published as a proposed rule in the May 3, 2007, Federal Register. Effective October 2008, CMS eliminated Medicare hospital reimbursement for the cost of eight complications of underlying conditions if they occur in the hospital. HHS anticipates the addition of more diagnoses to this "no-payment list" in the future. Programs designed to decrease the occurrence or to prevent these complications (e.g., policies, procedures) will likely result in a decreased incidence of these events at hospitals across the country.

## Health Care Quality Improvement Act and Peer Review Protection

Peer review is an activity whereby one health care professional examines the practice of another to determine competence in the practice of medicine. In the past, there were concerns about the potential for abuse of peer review, and peers were at risk of disclosure. Because such disclosure could result in costly and time-consuming litigation and/or potential damage to one's reputation, many physicians were dissuaded from participating in peer review.

The Health Care Quality Improvement Act (HCQIA) of 1986 (Title IV of Public Law No. 99-660) was created at a time when the number of malpractice cases was rising, with increasingly large settlements. Malpractice and the perceived risks of health care were in the public eye; the time was ripe for actions to ensure patient safely. Physicians reportedly considered early retirement and/or the elimination of certain procedures from their practices to reduce the risks and costs of malpractice. Oversight of physicians and other professionals (e.g., licensure, credentialing) was being strengthened, and peer review needed to be made safe for physicians.

Although the HCQIA resulted in peer review protection for institutions and individuals engaged in peer review, another major provision, the creation of the National Practitioner Data Bank (NPDB), was not realized until after publication of the final regulations in 1989. The database content was further amended by the 1990 Omnibus Budget Reconciliation Act (OBRA), which added a requirement that adverse determinations (findings and actions) by peer review of private accreditation entities should be reported to the NPDB.[8] A major provision of the HCQIA is the immunity provided to bodies that conduct peer review. Organizations covered under this act include hospitals, managed care organizations, professional societies, or committees of physicians at a national, state, or local level, which engaged in professional review activities through a formal peer review process. The expressed objective of these organizations should be to improve the quality of health care. The protection afforded by the act is "qualified immunity" from damages under state and federal law if the provisions of the act are followed (Table 9-1). The act relates to deliberations of professional bodies and actions taken as a result of the peer review process. Individuals who take part in these activities are also protected (see *Imperial v Suburban Hosp. Assn., Inc.*, 37 F3d 1026 [4th Cir 199]; *Decker v IHC Hospitals, Inc.*, 982 F2d 433 [10th Cir 1995]). The HCQIA establishes immunity from liability only, not immunity

---

TABLE 9-1   Requirements for the Peer Review Activities to Be Granted Immunity

1. The review and the resultant action must adversely affect the physician's clinical privileges and be based on clinical competence or conduct issues.

2. The action taken must be imposed with the reasonable belief that it will improve the quality of care.

3. The physician must be provided with due process rights within a specific time frame. The procedure for providing appeal rights and time frames are clearly stated in the act. The physicians must be made aware of the following:
   • The potential adverse action.
   • The basis for the action, the right to request a hearing (within not less than 30 days).
   • The hearing process and the witnesses to be called.
   • He or she can be represented by counsel and may cross-examine the witnesses and present evidence.
   • The hearing is to be recorded with the production of a written report, a copy of which is presented to the physicians.

Actions taken must be reported within a specified time frame to the data bank.

from suit. HCQIA also specifically denies immunity for claims alleging civil rights violations (42 USC §11111[b] professional review).

In the context of accusation of violation of civil rights, peer review protection can be pierced. In one civil rights case *Russell Adkins v Christie*, 488 F.3d 1324 (11th Cir 2007), a three-judge panel of the 11th U.S. Circuit Court of Appeals requested review of peer review records to investigate a potential civil rights violation. The physician alleged that an action had been taken based on his race. The court decided that rooting out "insidious discrimination" had priority over the need to keep private peer review deliberations secret. The judges ruled the information contained in the peer review was integral to the charge of racial discrimination, and Dr. Adkins had been subjected to a higher level of review, resulting in his termination of privileges.

Peer review cannot be used as a shield in cases where physicians are disciplined based on race, economic reasons (i.e., no reasonable belief that the review will improve quality of care), or failure to utilize appropriate peers (i.e., failure to demonstrate a reasonable effort was made to obtain and to review the facts related to the determination of an action).

Peer review protection is provided only if the objective of peer review is conducted in good faith with the prime objective of the activity to improve the quality of health care. The review and resultant action must adversely affect the physician's clinical privileges and be based in clinical competence or conduct issues. The process for appeals is specifically documented in the act. Table 9-2 lists a number of potential pitfalls to be avoided.

---

**TABLE 9-2    Challenges to Peer Review Immunity**

Challenges may be made to the immunity of the deliberations by allegation of "sham peer review" or peer review being conducted in bad faith if:

- The physician is not made aware of the potential adverse action and the basis for the action.
- Procedural requirements were not met (i.e., the physician is not provided his due process rights, and a fair hearing was not offered).
- The required time frames for the hearing were not met.
- The physician is not informed that s(he) may be represented by an attorney.
- The physician is not made aware of the hearing process and the witnesses to be called.
- The physician is not offered the ability to cross-examine witnesses and present evidence.
- The physician was not provided with a copy of the report.
- The case related is to a civil rights claim.
- The action was taken to decrease competition (e.g., collusion between members of the peer review panel who were direct competitors of the physician under review).
- Actions were not taken with the main objective to improve care, but to remove a troublesome staff member or to silence a "malcontent" or whistle blower.

Immunity depends on adherence to requirements including time frames, notification, and procedural issues.

## The National Practitioner Data Bank

Instituted in 1990, the NPDB[9] collects data that include the following:

- Professional review actions taken by hospitals, HMOs, and other entities that result in reduction, suspension, revoking of clinical privileges, restriction, or termination of privileges or membership in a health care entity. Any action that adversely affects the clinical privileges of a physician for a period longer than 30 days must be reported.

- Acceptance of the surrender of clinical privileges or restriction of privileges while the physician is under investigation by the health care entity concerning issues of incompetence or improper professional conduct, or as an alternative to conducting an investigation.

- Professional board actions that result in a change in licensure status.

- Exclusion from Medicare–Medicaid programs; sanctions.

- Malpractice payments and settlements made on behalf of physicians.

The HCQIA (§ 11135 Title 42, Chapter 117, Subchapter II, Duty of Hospitals) creates the expectation that hospitals will use the NPDB contents for credentialing. The information will be available to other entities, including managed care organizations. It is an expectation that the NPDB will be queried by a hospital at the time a physician applies for credentialing for a position on its medical staff, including courtesy status, and every subsequent 2 years (the expected interval for recredentialing). As noted in the Act, "Any hospital which does not request the information (for review) as required in paragraph (a) of this section is presumed to have knowledge of any information reported to the Data Bank. . . ."[10]

The HCQIA specifically states who may have access to the Data Bank, including the following:[11]

1. A hospital that requests information concerning a physician, dentist, or other health care practitioner who is on its medical staff (courtesy or otherwise) or has clinical privileges at the hospital;
2. A physician, dentist, or other health care practitioner, who requests information concerning himself or herself;
3. Boards of Medical Examiners or other State licensing boards;

4. Health care entities which have entered or may be entering employment or affiliation relationships with a physician, dentist or other health care practitioner, or to which the physician, dentist, or other health care practitioner has applied for clinical privileges or appointment to the medical staff;

5. An attorney, or individual representing himself or herself, who has filed a medical malpractice action or claim in a State or Federal court or other adjudicative body against a hospital, and who requests information regarding a specific physician, dentist, or other health care practitioner who is also named in the action or claim, provided that this information will be disclosed only upon the submission of evidence that the hospital failed to request information from the Data Bank as required by Sec. 60.10(a), and may be used solely with respect to litigation resulting from the action or claim against the hospital;

6. A health care entity with respect to professional review activity.

Practitioners may dispute the accuracy of the content of the report within 60 days from the date on which the report was mailed. There are specific instructions in the act as to what actions can be taken to dispute an entry. HCQIA allows the U.S. Department of Health and Human Services (HHS) to promulgate regulations that allow a health care practitioner to challenge information reported to HHS (42 USC §11136[2]).

State boards and health care entities who participate in peer review activities are to report disciplinary actions they have taken to the NPDB.

## HIPAA and Its Multiple Titles

Public Law 104-191, HIPAA, was designed to address multiple aspects of health care and has different rules that became effective at different times. The Act had two titles: Title I was Health Care Access, Portability, and Renewability; and Title II was Preventing Health Care Fraud and Abuse, Administrative Simplification, and Medical Liability Reform (Table 9-3).

**TABLE 9-3  Multiple Titles of the Health Insurance Portability and Accountability Act**

**Title I** addresses issues related to health care access, portability of insurance coverage, and issues related to health insurance affected by change or loss of employment. It prevented group health plans eligibility and/or premium adjustments being based on health status, medical history, or disability. These protections, which have qualifications, were not offered to private individual insurance.

**Title II** was responsible for the creation of specific rules related to privacy, transactions and code sets, security, unique identifiers, and enforcement.

## The Privacy Rule

This rule is comprised of regulations that govern the use in disclosure of protected health information (PHI), either in electronic or paper form. PHI is any health-related information, health status, and information relating to health care provisions, payment, and any information contained in the medical record. Specific exceptions to this rule include reporting to law enforcement officials evidence of child abuse and reporting infectious disease. The key to disclosure of PHI between health professionals is that the minimum amount of information necessary should be released. Covered entities (defined in the rule[12] as those who are "covered by the regulations") must also track release of this PHI and must designate an individual to be responsible for educating all staff on the Privacy Rule and overseeing the confidentiality provisions of HIPAA. Covered entities are required to have designated privacy officers and policies and procedures used to educate the facility or office staff and to ensure compliance with the act.

The Privacy Rule gives the patient the right to review his/her medical record and to correct any errors. The covered entity can disclose information as part of ongoing treatment, payment during normal operations of the facility or office, and if authorized by the patient. The privacy officer is responsible for ensuring that these privacy activities occur consistently, in addition to ensuring compliance with other HIPAA requirements. Upon initially accessing care, patients are provided with a privacy notice (i.e., an explanation of the organization's use of information and the patient's rights regarding its use and release of the information contained in the medical records). The patient's acknowledgment of receipt of this information must be retained.

## The Transactions and Code Sets Rule

This rule mandated the simplification of data collection and aggregation through the creation of universal data sets and the fostering of interoperability of programs, including electronic data interchange functions. Common codes have the following advantages:[13]

- Facilitating electronic filing of health claims
- Decreasing costs of electronic interactions in the long term
- Decreasing the errors that result in rejected claims
- Providing a more universal system for data collection and interoperability between various systems and programs, including claim adjudication of health data collection
- Improving transparency related to the delivery of health care

## Facilitated Health Care Fraud and Abuse Investigation and Reporting

Defined and identified here are fraud and abuse offenses. Also created was an additional database for collecting information listed below. These data sets could also be data mined to identify circumstances that lead to increased risk of fraud and abuse.

*The Healthcare Integrity and Protection Data Bank (HIPDB)*
The HIPDB[11] collects reports on final adverse actions including the following:

1. Civil judgments from federal and state courts related to the provisions of goods and services, findings against health care providers and suppliers, actions taken by federal or state agencies against health care providers and suppliers related to licensing and certification

2. Exclusion from participation in federal or state health care programs

3. Federal or state criminal convictions against health suppliers and providers

*The Security Rule*
The Security Rule consists of security safeguards for electronic PHI. As part of HIPAA, a unique identifier was created for all covered entities using EDI. This national provider identifier (NPI) will replace all other identifiers including the unique provider identification number (UPIN).

*The Enforcement Rule*
The Enforcement Rule, issued in 2006, sets penalties for violations of HIPAA rules and creates a structure for investigations and hearings related to violations.

## Medical Errors and Transparency

A number of industry groups actively encourage acknowledging medical errors, especially those that are apparent to the patient–family and those that do not result in harm. The National Quality Forum (NQF) supports disclosure of this information as a practice that promotes safe care.[14] In 2001, the Joint Commission issued a nationwide disclosure statement requiring that patients be made aware of all outcomes of care. A number of major hospitals and health systems support acknowledging errors, providing an apology, explaining how the error could have happened, and communicating the action that will be taken to prevent a recurrence in the future.

The VA Medical Center in Lexington, Kentucky, has had a full disclosure policy since the 1980s.[15,16] The University of Illinois Medical Center (UIC)[16] has a well-known error disclosure program and a specific curriculum to train medical students to recognize medical errors, deal with the repercussions, and know what actions to take. Since 2001, when it began to acknowledge medical mistakes and negotiate settlements with injured patients, the University of Michigan Health System has experienced a significant decrease in the number of pending malpractice claims.[17] Although a majority of states now have "apology laws" that prevent expressions of regret from being used in a malpractice suit, there are individuals and organizations that continue to doubt the robustness of these laws.

The IOM report *To Err Is Human: Building a Safer Health System* highlighted the issue of medical errors and recommended the NQF as the entity to develop reporting standards, error reporting requirements for health care organizations, and nonpunitive reporting systems.[6]

Medical ethics supports truth telling. A risk management approach that advocates reporting errors to patients believes that transparency will result in fewer lawsuits, early settlements, better understanding of the systemic source of errors, and the diffusing of anger through early communication. Leading clinical journals contain articles relating to disclosure to patients, and there is a growing body of knowledge in this area (e.g., a framework for apologies, how to frame the admission, and the right time and place for an apology).[15-19]

A number of state governments have pursued disclosure-related legislation. For example, a Pennsylvania law contains time frames for disclosure and a prohibition for use of this communication as evidence of liability in litigation. Although more than 30 states have some sort of apology law protecting expressions of regret and apologies from being used in litigation, these have not been tested sufficiently to provide a sense of safety to physicians, attorneys, and insurance companies. As noted in a *New England Journal of Medicine* review article ("Disclosing Harmful Medical Errors to Patients") "plaintiffs' attorneys, who must sift through dozens of prospective claims in choosing which ones to pursue, will prize information gained from disclosures, whether or not they are permitted to use that information as evidence in subsequent litigation."[16 (p.2716)]

A national coalition of patients, attorneys, physicians, and hospital administrators—the Sorry Works! Coalition—has proposed that hospital staff review all adverse events and that hospital administrators and physicians institute a dialogue with patients and families to explain what happened, apologize for any errors committed, and offer fair compensation.[15]

The authors of a January–February 2007 *Health Affairs* article titled "Disclosure of Medical Injury to Patients: An Improbable Risk Management Strategy" have a different perspective on the financial impact of the trend toward full disclosure.[19] They posit that any decrease in the number and the amount of claims deferred due to apologies and admitting errors may be offset by the increase in patient awareness of medical errors. Adverse outcomes once attributed to expected results of diseases or therapies are now acknowledged as medical errors and, as such, the responsibility of the clinician. There is a widespread belief that the vast majority of medical errors do not result in litigation or suits, and it remains to be seen if identifying more errors and bringing them to the patient's attention will decrease the rate or impact of malpractice litigation.

## Basics of Malpractice

Medical malpractice and the problems associated with it remain an important issue in the U.S. medical community. The general concept of professional malpractice can be traced to English legal theory as early as the 14th century; however, it was not until the mid-19th century that it began to be applied in real-world situations.[5,20,21] Today, an American doctor has a greater chance of being sued than any other doctor in the world. While some feel that it serves to "weed out bad doctors," malpractice also can adversely affect physicians who practice within the standards of reasonable care.

*Medical malpractice* is an act or omission by a health care provider that deviates from accepted standards of practice in the medical community and that causes harm or injury to the patient. Fear of malpractice results in the practice of defensive medicine, which may put patients at risk for unnecessary treatments and testing and may further deplete limited resources. Concerns about malpractice may hinder open clinical quality management activities (e.g., access to quality management documents may be limited due to the fear of releasing potentially damaging information).[21]

Negligence is the most common cause for malpractice cases wherein the defendant–physician is accused of failing to exercise due care. In the majority of these cases, four specific elements are required to prove negligence. These elements are listed in Table 9-4.

*Clinical practice guidelines* (CPGs) are used by attorneys for both the defense and the plaintiff to demonstrate that a standard of care has, or has not, been met. In a malpractice trial, guidelines are weighted on the basis of the issuing body, the purpose of the guideline, and evidence of peer review of the CPG. For instance, managed care organizations' utilization-based guidelines are weighted differently than clinical medical society guidelines, which are created with reference to evidence-based medicine or expert consensus. While CPGs may be used as a "reference," the jury decides how to weigh their content based on expert witnesses' testimonies. In the case of *Frakes v Cardiology Consultants, P.C.* (1997 WL 536949, Tenn Cir App [1997]), the court considered a table,

---

### TABLE 9-4  Elements of Negligence

**A duty to treat:**
Based on the existence of a patient–physician contractual relationship to provide care at the level of an average physician. Proving that action was legally required.

**Breach of duty to provide average care:**
Physicians are required to provide reasonable and ordinary care, skill, and diligence as other physicians with the same area of practice. Physicians testify in court as expert witnesses to define the standard of care of a physician in this specialty area or practice.

Experts who testify are usually of the same specialty or have appropriate education and experience similar to the physician accused of malpractice. Practice guidelines have been referred to as standards of care, especially nationally recognized standards.

**Causation:**
The outcome would not have occurred but for the physician's action or failure to act. The proximate cause is not required to be the sole cause of the action, but only a significant factor.

**Evidence of injury–damages:**
Evidence of harm.

"Exercise Test Parameters Associated with Poor Prognosis and/or Increased Severity of CAD" contained in American College of Cardiology and American Heart Association brochures as a consensus statement on the interpretation of an exercise treadmill test based on the fact that all the experts adopted the document as the correct standard of care. In contrast, in *Liberatore v Kaufman* (835 So2d 404, Fla App [2003]), the Florida Court of Appeals held that the trial court had abused its discretion when it used a bulletin published by the American College of Obstetricians and Gynecologists to bolster the testimony of their expert witness. Practice guidelines have also been used to impeach expert testimony (*Roper v Blumenfeld* 309 NJ Super 219 [1998]). In general, an accepted clinical standard may be presumptive evidence of due care, but expert testimony is required to introduce the standard and to establish its source and relevancy.

The standard of proof imposed by judges in a malpractice suit is less stringent than the "beyond a reasonable doubt" standard used in criminal trials, and the concept of contributory negligence is considered in awarding damages. The contribution of the patient's actions or inactions that resulted in the injury is also noted (i.e., did the patient act as a "reasonable, prudent person" would have given his condition). If the patient failed to follow the physician's clear and documented instructions, to report a change in symptoms, or to fill or take a prescription, he or she might be found partially responsible, and the final award would be lessened. Failure by the physician to provide follow-up care or to provide and document instructions may serve as proof that the physician is at least partially responsible. Handwriting legibility, evidence of adequate informed consent, and adequate delivery of specific discharge information also may have a significant impact on the outcome of litigation.

There are other legal pitfalls in providing medical care and overseeing quality (e.g., incorrect or inadequate informed consent prior to a surgical intervention can result in a charge of assault or battery).[5] The physician and risk managers must be aware that if a procedure is changed without patient permission, or if additional surgery occurs without adequate informed consent, the physician may be at risk for litigation.

Cases of infectious disease require special attention. Patients must be made aware of their communicability and the actions that must be taken to prevent the spread of disease to others. Suits brought by sexual partners in various states have resulted in decisions that held physicians liable for the spread of HIV (e.g., physicians have been held responsible for providing and for documenting advice given to the patient to prevent the spread of the disease). In the case of *Reisner v Regents of University of California* (31 Cal App 4th 1195 [1995]), the court held that a sexual partner of a patient had a cause of action against the patient's physician and the hospital for failing to inform the patient that she had been contaminated with HIV-infected blood and was at risk of spreading the disease. The ruling stated that the physician and the hospital had a duty to counsel and to educate the patient on how to prevent the spread of the virus.

If malpractice is proven, there are two types of damages: compensatory and punitive. *Compensatory damages* compensate the patient for past and future cost, pain, anguish, and loss of income. The intent is to restore that patient to the condition he or she was in prior to the incident. Monetary compensation is awarded to approximate the harm caused.

*Punitive damages* are a means for the judicial system to "send a message" and financially punish a defendant. Juries award punitive damages, sometimes in the millions of dollars, as punishment for willful or malicious conduct. The tobacco litigation settlement is an example of punitive damages (because sanctions were imposed to punish the defendant).

## Facility–Organizational Risk Management Issues

Managed care organizations, hospitals, and other facilities have been held liable for harm to patients through alleged failure to use reasonable care to ensure the competency of their providers upon credentialing and recredentialing and/or to have an appropriate number of competent medical and support staff (*Darling v Charleston Community Memorial Hospital*, 33 Ill2d 326, 211 NE2d 253, 14 ALR3d 860 [Ill 1965]).

The doctrine of corporate negligence holds that an organization has an independent duty to the patient in credentialing its personnel. An organization may also be sued on the basis of services provided to the facility by independent contractors. For example, emergency services delivered by a contracted emergency room (ER) group may expose the facility to litigation on the basis of the legal concepts of vicarious liability and ostensible or apparent agency. In such cases, the patient came to the hospital seeking care and the institution or hospital appeared to present the contract ER physician as its employee. In a similar manner, a private anesthesiologist may appear to be an extension of the facility and thus incur liability for poor outcomes or adverse events under a legal theory of ostensible agency. Although the contract between the facility and the treatment group may allocate liability, the patient may be inclined to name all likely parties in the litigation.

Liability due to failure to exercise appropriate care is not limited to individual practitioners. It can involve the chief of clinical areas, the chief medical officers, and other officers of the corporate suite. The concept of the surgeon as "captain of the ship" in the OR holds that the physician is responsible for the actions of his or her subordinates. The legal concept of *respondeat superior* (Latin for "let the master answer") holds the employer responsible for the actions of employees. A health plan or a hospital also may be sued for the actions of their employees. This is known as *vicarious liability*.

Adequate credentialing is required, for example, querying the NPDB and HIPDB as suggested in the HCQIA, and following procedures and policies embodied in leading health care accreditors. Hospitals and other facilities have been sued for failing to exercise reasonable care in credentialing participating specialists (e.g., *Harrell v Total Health Care*, 781 SW2d 58 [MO 1989]). Pivotal cases have clearly stated that organizations are responsible for utilization review actions and their impact on the care provided (see *Wickline v State of California*, 192 Cal App 3d 1630, 239 Cal Rptr 810 [Ct App 1986] and *Fox v Health Net*, Riverside Sup Ct Case No 219692 [1993]).

Bad faith action suits can be brought against managed care organizations and their staff related to utilization management activities (i.e., for failure to promptly and to adequately review requests for care, for failure to provide timely approval of care, and for failure to provide expedited reviews for cases as required in organization requirements or as imposed by state or federal law).

## Antitrust in Medicine

Antitrust issues arise when a significant number of individuals who provide a service work together to control how the goods or services are provided or distributed (i.e., controlling reimbursement rates or access). This can present a potential risk when market players, health systems, or a number of individuals work together (even if ostensibly for the purpose of improving how care is provided) and when they create and enforce clinical guidelines that influence how providers practice medicine for a specific clinical condition. The Sherman Antitrust Act (July 2, 1890, ch 647, 26 Stat 209, 15 USC §1-7), refers to "contracts or combinations in restraint of trade" (§1). The act includes actions taken together in a given market to engage in intended "parallel conduct" or fee setting (i.e., sharing of pricing information).

Other sections of the act relate to unilateral actions of a single business in an attempt to monopolize a market. Cases involve hospital and managed care organizations but can occur at the medical group level. A recent case was brought against two clinics for refusing to accept new Medicaid members and possibly collaborating in this decision. The Sherman Act can be violated by agreements among provider-controlled networks and plans when competing physicians set, by majority vote, the maximum fees that they may claim in full payment for health services provided to policyholders of specified insurance plans (*Arizona v Maricopa County Medical Society*, 457 US 332 [1982]). Similar issues may arise as multiple medical groups of managed care organizations come together to write common guidelines that restrain reimbursement for certain treatments and exclude other possible treatments.

Regarding the issue of cartels and professionalism, the Federal Trade Commission (FTC) has successfully challenged provider cartels that engage in a wide variety of practices designed to raise prices, to limit competition from other providers, or to affect the cost containment efforts of managed care organizations. In the case of *United States v North Dakota Hospital Association* (640 F Supp 1028 [DND 1986]), the issue revolved around hospitals' joint refusal to extend discounts in bidding for contracts.

Groups and associations can run afoul of antitrust law through restrictions on advertising and dissemination of information (*California Dental Association v Federal Trade Commission*, 526 US 756 [1999]). FTC jurisdiction extends to associations (e.g., the California Dental Association) that provide substantial economic benefit to its for-profit members. Private accreditation and professional standard settings can risk antitrust suits for conducting or for recommending boycotts or other actions that would result in the restraint of trade or for giving an unfair advantage to one group over another. The case of

*Wilk v American Medical Association* (895 F2d 352 [2d Cir 1990]) affirmed the District Court's finding that the American Medical Association violated the Sherman Act by conducting an illegal boycott in restraint of trade directed at chiropractors.

When payers with "market power" take actions related to reimbursement it is not always considered antitrust. In the case of *Kartell v Blue Shield of Mass.* (749 F2d 922 1st Cir [1984]), Blue Shield's ban on "balanced billing" was not considered a violation of the Sherman Act.

The crafting of clinical guidelines and the advent of pay-for-performance programs (P4P) have exposed more potential risks for running afoul of antitrust law. The AHRQ points out the risks of antitrust when crafting P4P programs in its guide, *Pay-for-Performance: A Decision Guide for Purchasers.*[22] This guide references the *Antitrust Guidelines for Collaborations Among Competitors* issued by the FTC and the U.S. Department of Justice in April, 2000. The article suggests that antitrust counsel should be consulted if payers are considering collaborating, particularly regarding payment/provider contracting issues,[23] and recommends the creation and/or adoption of uniform P4P quality or performance standards.

## Alternative Dispute Resolution: Arbitration–Mediation

With the issues of litigation, the increase in malpractice suits and settlements, and the time frame involved in depositions and preparation for a suit and court dates, forms of alternative dispute resolution are gaining in popularity. Arbitration is one example of an alternative to a malpractice trial. Arbiters are considered to be more knowledgeable of issues and less biased than a lay jury, and the proceedings are more private. Arbiters may act singly or as part of a panel. Deliberations are usually shorter and less stressful than a trial, and there is direct dialogue between the two parties. Some malpractice carriers offer discounts to physicians who have their patients sign arbitration agreements. Unlike malpractice trials, which may be taken by an attorney on contingency, the patient may be required to pay the arbiter, the experts, a lawyer, and other fees. Rulings do not allow for appeal rights.

*Arbitration* is used when the parties agree to have a third party decide on the merits of a claim. The single arbiter or panel allocates blame and may impose an award for damages much like a court. The process is streamlined due to the lack of a jury and/or many expert witnesses. While practicing physicians may have an office policy to request that patients sign an agreement consenting to binding arbitration if an issue arises, questions have arisen concerning the patient's understanding that, by signing the agreement, they are signing away their right to a jury trial.

Physicians generally prefer "alternative dispute" systems. There is the perception that these processes are less expensive, less time-consuming, and may result in decreasing the rate of malpractice premiums. Arbitration can be either mandatory or voluntary. Some states mandate arbitration prior to the commencement of a malpractice suit to lessen court time and to facilitate resolution of the dispute without lengthy litigation. Benefits of arbitration include the following: it may be less confrontational and less costly; it may include written expert opinion without the added expense and time or witnesses; and it may include an agreement to keep the hearing and the settlement confidential.

*Mediation* is a form of conflict resolution that brings two or more parties together to discuss their issues with the assistance of a mediator (an impartial third party), but does not involve a binding decision. Mediation usually begins as an airing of grievances after which the mediator attempts to have the parties come to a settlement with the mediator acting as an "honest broker." The mediator has no power to require a settlement.

In 2003, CMS directed its program (Quality Improvement Organization [QIO]) to create a free, nationwide mediation program as an alternative to a quality review process initiated by a beneficiary complaint.[24] The quality review process used as the primary investigational method for beneficiary complaints was seen by some as a slow, time-consuming program that was confrontational rather than collaborative and that did not result in improved communications between the providers and beneficiaries, especially in areas of the following:

- Complaints concerning quality of services
- Communication issues
- Quality of care issues from the beneficiaries' perspective

Participation in mediation is voluntary, and the mediation request must be initiated by the beneficiary. Mediators do not make decisions or influence the outcome of the mediation. Both the beneficiary and the physician, provider, or facility representative must agree to participate, and the dialogue can be terminated by either party at any time. Mediations can be conducted in a safe, neutral environment or over the telephone. Each party has an opportunity to tell his/her story, to express concerns directly to the physician (or other provider of health care services), and to listen to the response. With the approval of both parties, the beneficiary and/or physician may bring a lawyer to act in the capacity of an advisor.

A typical mediation session takes between 2 and 4 hours. The key to this process is that the patient drives the system and controls how the complaint is resolved. If a mutual resolution is reached, the QIO will follow up and monitor the terms of the agreement. This process can address issues that are not contained in the medical record and facilitate explanations between patients and health care providers.

Some types of cases are not appropriate for mediation (e.g., gross and flagrant quality of care issues and cases already in litigation). Mediation sessions are not recorded; any written notes taken during the mediation are destroyed at the end of the session. Parties to the mediation agree not to use information uncovered during the mediation in any future legal proceedings. If the parties reach a resolution, an agreement may be drafted and signed, concluding the mediation session. Federal and state laws protect the confidentiality of mediation sessions, per the Federal Rule of Evidence (Article IV) 408.[25] Many U.S. District Courts and Courts of Appeal have court rules providing for the confidentiality of mediation negotiations. (i.e., US Ct of App 4th Cir Rule 33), and many states specifically provide for the confidentiality of statements and documents used in mediation.

# Ethics

Beauchamp and Childress list "respect for autonomy, beneficence and non-maleficence, and justice" as the main principles of bioethics and the basic foundations for many ethical prescriptions and evaluations of human actions.[26 (p.398)] Application of these principles was recommended with consideration to requirements such as validity, value of the research, fair patient participation, favorable risk-benefit ratio, informed consent, and independent review.

## Respect for Autonomy

*Autonomy*, a deliberate self-decision, emphasizes an individual's capability to determine his/her personal goals. It serves as the keystone for patients' participation in their own health care decisions and for the present-day emphasis on informed consent. Under this principle, a patient who is competent makes his/her choice as to whether or not to engage in the treatment options presented. Patients who are competent have the capacity to make a judgment based on their understanding of their medical condition and the impact of failing to undergo a recommended treatment or test. Some patients make decisions that the physician feels are wrong or not in their best interest (e.g., leaving a hospital against medical advice).

Informed consent requires that the patient clearly understand the decision he or she is making and the potential risks and benefits of the decision. Asking the patient to repeat back the information communicated is one method for determining patient understanding of the content of a communication. A patient who does not demonstrate the ability to understand the issue may be unable to exercise autonomy, and a substitute decision-maker may need to be identified.

## Beneficence and Nonmaleficence

This principle aims to improve patient care and safety by advocating the principle "do no harm." It focuses on maximizing potential benefit while minimizing harm and risk to the patient. QI projects that incorporate the principle of beneficence go beyond the patient's medical needs and include elements of compassion and kindness. Guided by this ethical principle, QI must aim to do no harm, to maximize benefits, and to minimize harm to secure the well-being of patients.

## Justice

The ethical principle of justice encompasses concepts such as equal access to care, provision of treatment and resources according to need, fair distribution of health care benefits and burdens, good stewardship of an organization's and a society's resources, and accountability. The benefits and burdens of research participation must be distributed equitably, and IRBs play a key role in ensuring subject selection is equitable. The principle of justice also implies that a benefit to which a person is entitled should not be denied without good reason or when some burden is imposed unduly.

## CASE STUDY ● ● ●

### Clinical Quality and Patient Autonomy

QI relates not only to the quality of clinical care provided, but also to patient choice and autonomy. Mary Elizabeth Wainwright, a lifetime smoker, had lived in a high-rise senior citizen residence for 27 years. At age 93, she had outlived her husband, her son, and all her relatives. She was brought to the ER by ambulance, mentally alert but severely short of breath. Her pulmonary condition had deteriorated, and she had been ventilator dependent for the past 2 months. She was a favorite on the chronic vent unit, always smiling. The only problem for the staff was that she kept pulling at her endotracheal tube and telling everyone that she wanted the staff to let her die. Although attempts to wean her from the ventilator failed, the staff continued to try a "slow wean."

The hospital had difficulty finding a chronic vent unit to take Mary because of recently diagnosed brittle diabetes, severe rheumatoid arthritis, and ischemic cardiomyopathy.

The intern stated to the nursing staff, "This is a futile case. Why not shut off the ventilator and let nature take its course? The money could be better spent elsewhere."

The hospital risk manager was concerned that honoring the patient's wishes might result in a long-lost relative suing the hospital. The attending physician did not believe that anyone would choose to die. "She must be delusional . . . I won't obey a crazy person's wishes."

Confused about what to do, the senior resident calls a member of the ethics committee for advice. Before the ethics committee meets, a member of the committee meets with the patient. The patient communicates the following: "I have lived a long life and liked best to walk around, watering my plants and talking to my cat. All my friends and relatives have died. My eyesight and hearing are rapidly failing, and my joints hurt from being in bed so long." She stated that she expected more pain in the future, without significant improvement. She did not expect to be taken off the respirator or to walk around her apartment ever again. She had lived long enough and therefore chose to die.

The ethics committee met with the attending physician, resident, intern, and key nursing staff. The committee member who spoke with Mrs. Wainwright provided the patient's rationale and discussed the patient's wishes and her capacity to make a decision of this magnitude. The committee reviewed the concepts of nonmaleficence, beneficence, and autonomy. Options were discussed with emphasis on how to best serve the patient's interests.

### Discussion

This case touches on a number of ethical principles. If a treatment involves pain, repeated hospital visits, lab tests, or prolonged hospitalization, the physician may still choose maximizing lifespan. However, maximizing lifespan may not have the same utility for an elderly patient who values freedom from pain and suffering or an escape from a prolonged final decline in a hospital. Compassion and the requirements of informed consent enable patients to make decisions based on their desires and personal values.

Mrs. Wainwright was subsequently evaluated by a psychiatrist who found no evidence of psychiatric illness that would affect her decision-making capacity. She was informed about her condition, and she demonstrated a good understanding of her current situation (i.e., it was highly unlikely that she would be weaned from the ventilator, and she was severely limited in what she could do). She saw her life as ongoing suffering without happiness. She made a rational decision based on her assessment of the situation and her values.

Advance directives, a living will, or health care power of attorney would not apply in this case because the patient was capable of making her own decisions. Continuing her life would not provide happiness or satisfaction and could be seen as causing psychic and physical harm. Providing medications to relieve pain would likely cause sedation and respiratory depression. These concepts were discussed with the staff.

The staff discussed the patient's choice of termination of life support with her one final time, and she remained adamant. She was given a low dose of morphine as needed for her unremitting arthritis pain, and her weekly weaning began the next morning as scheduled. The staff made sure that she was kept comfortable during the weaning attempt and supported her request not to be placed back on the respirator.

Harm was prevented (nonmaleficence) by discontinuing futile care that prolonged the patient's suffering. It was the concept of beneficence that allowed the patient to exert autonomy in choosing life or death after being fully informed of her prognosis. Not returning the patient to the respirator had the highest utility for her.

Since the late 1960s, health care ethics has undergone a shift from beneficence and professional authority to patient centeredness as a result of the Federal Patient Self-Determination Act, an amendment to the Omnibus Budget Reconciliation Act of 1990. The act, which took effect on December 1, 1991, mandated that patients receive information about end-of-life care and their right to draft advance directives. *Advance directives* are documents that express a patient's health care choices or name another person to make decisions regarding medical treatment in the event that the patient is unable to make these decisions themselves. Advance directives are composed of a living will, a power of attorney, and a health care proxy.

## Human Subjects Research and QI

A sound study design is central to any human subjects research. The overall study design must ensure that the study question can be clearly answered and that risks to participants can be minimized in proportion to the benefits.[27,28] Risk may be physical, psychological, social, and/or economic, and many potential subjects may be excluded from a study because their condition, their ability to communicate, or other factors put them at higher risk.

QI is defined as methodical, data-guided activities designed to bring about positive changes in the delivery of health care in local settings.[22] Most urgently needed QI activity focuses on changing practices that result in suboptimal care. Landmark reports on medical errors by IOM have resulted in national initiatives to improve the quality of health care delivery, and recent advances in health care quality and the practice of QI have generated discussion about the ethics of QI.[6,7]

Ethical discussions pertaining to QI increased when a physician published results of a QI project.[29] The project, conducted by the End Stage Renal Disease Network, was accepted by CMS as QI; however, the Office of Human Research Protection (OHRP) ruled that the project was research and required oversight by the IRB. This led to concerns among clinicians that their efforts to conduct patient-related QI projects could be construed as a violation of regulations.

In 2002, the Hastings Center undertook a project focused on distinguishing QI from research and published a report with recommendations for change.[28] Simultaneously, several health care delivery and research organizations met to discuss ethical oversight for their QI initiatives. The details of this discussion appear in the 2006 Hastings Center Report.[28]

---

## CASE STUDY • • •

### Is It Research or QI?

In 2004, the University of Texas initiated a clinical quality project aimed at increasing adherence to standard heart failure medications at discharge, based on a CMS project for chronic care hospitals. The project aimed to achieve adherence greater than 90% of the time. This multidisciplinary collaborative project involved experts from various disciplines. Experts with research backgrounds viewed the project as a research study designed to increase adherence through interventions and recommended IRB approval. Experts with a clinical background viewed it as a project to improve clinical quality for patients by adhering to national standards (i.e., a component of clinical practice and operations). After several meetings and discussions, the clinical quality group reviewed existing literature on the topic and found that such confusion existed across the nation.

---

## Institutional Review Boards

IRBs came into being in the early 1970s when the Department of Health, Education, and Welfare issued regulations that reflected the NIH's Policies for the Protection of Human Subjects. IRBs are focused on evaluating and on approving human subject research through the use of the informed consent process that stipulates for individual participants the associated risks and benefits, including the right to refuse to participate and the right to withdraw. Ethical principles are utilized to define actions that are right and wrong based on available scientific information and patient wishes.

The challenge in clinical research is deciding between the lesser of two evils or the greater of two goods. Principles and applications of these ethical issues in oversight for human research are discussed extensively by the OHRP for clinical research in the *Belmont Report*[30] and other published reports.[31]

IRBs are mandated by federal law to protect the rights and the welfare of human subjects participating in research using a peer review method. An IRB, also known as an independent ethics committee (IEC) or ethical review board (ERB), consists of a group of experts–scientists who are formally designated to evaluate, to approve, to monitor, and to review clinical, biomedical, epidemiological, and behavioral research involving humans with the aim to protect the rights and the welfare of the subjects. The HHS and the Food and Drug Administration (FDA) have empowered IRBs to evaluate research protocols based on scientific, legal, and ethical principles and to recommend approval, to require modifications, or to disapprove research projects as appropriate.

An IRB performs critical oversight functions for research conducted on human subjects that are scientific, ethical, and regulatory. HIPAA privacy regulations require an IRB to protect the privacy rights of research subjects in specific ways. At some health care organizations, the IRB reviews all HIPAA-required authorizations and waivers of authorizations for research use of identifiable health information.

In the United States, IRBs are governed by Title 45 CFR (Code of Federal Regulations) Part 46. This Research Act of 1974 defines IRBs and requires them for all research that receives direct or indirect funding from the department of HHS. IRBs are regulated by the Office for Human Research Protections within HHS.

IRBs were created in response to research abuses earlier in the 20th century. The risks of human experimentation came to public attention based on evidence presented at the Nuremberg trials concerning the inhumane treatment of participants in medical experiments by World War II Nazi doctors. The 1945 Nuremberg Code was the first legal attempt to deal with ethical issues of clinical research.[32] It encompasses principles of informed consent, absence of coercion, adhering to scientific principles, and beneficence toward experiment participants.

The 1964 Declaration of Helsinki resulted in a set of ethical principles for human experimentation being developed by the World Medical Association.[33] The declaration focused on informed consent but allowed surrogate consent for special situations (e.g., when a participant is incompetent or a minor), and encompassed risk benefit analysis, scientific experiments, and ethics review. The first significant effort by the medical community to regulate itself, the declaration led to formal ethical review processes such as IRB, IEC, and/or ERB.

Exploitation of human participants in the United States is best exemplified by the Tuskegee Syphilis Study, which involved 600 Black men—399 with syphilis, 201 without the disease—and was conducted between 1932 and 1972.[34] The *Tuskegee Study of Untreated Syphilis in the Negro Male* was designed to record the natural history of syphilis in hopes of justifying treatment programs for Blacks. Conducted without the benefit of patients' informed consent, participants with the disease were told that they were receiving treatment when, in fact, treatment was being withheld. Public awareness of this unethical study provided the impetus for the National Research Act and the creation of the National Commission for the Protection of Human Subjects of Biomedical and Behavioral Research, which defined ethical principles for research. The *Belmont Report*,[30] which followed, highlighted respect, beneficence, and justice. It continues to be an essential reference for IRBs.

To ensure patient autonomy, medical specialty societies, including the American College of Medical Quality (ACMQ), have developed policies related to experimental and investigational medical services and supplies. In the case of the ACMQ (policy no. 29),[35] research of experimental and investigational treatments must always be reviewed and approved by qualified experts, and patients' informed consents should be received before enrolling them in a study.

## Future Trends

The growing acceptance of apologies in medicine will likely have an impact on legal activity in this area. The risks and benefits of transparency will also become clearer in the next decade. The potential of a no-fault approach to malpractice may also significantly impede the growth in litigation that was observed at the end of the 20th century.

Patient safety and the protection afforded reporting entities, based on regulations and statutes, will also affect this area of quality improvement and the willingness of individuals and institutions to report adverse events. The impact of IRB requirements for QI projects and the potential impact of HIPAA on research projects will need to be resolved to prevent a slowing of progress in the field of QI and patient safety. Governmental intervention and/or legal action will greatly affect these issues over the next decade.

P4P and reporting data on care quality are two of the most widely advocated strategies for improving health care quality. Proponents of P4P argue that such programs could help improve the quality of care and deter the rate of growth in health care costs. Indeed, P4P systems have been implemented by some managed care plans that cover Medicaid beneficiaries, and proposals for establishing P4P systems for Medicare services continue to come before Congress. However, support for such a reward system is not universal. Paying physicians to provide care and to perform activities for which they are being reimbursed is seen by some as unethical, and, as a process, P4P may be difficult to implement.

## References

1. Wikipedia. Third Dynasty of Ur. http://en.wikipedia.org/wiki/Ur_III. Accessed July 31, 2008.
2. King LW. *The Code of Hammurabi.* Whitefish, MT: Kessinger Publishing; 2004.
3. Hippocrates. *Encyclopedia Britannica.* http://www.britannica.com/EBchecked/topic/266627/Hippocrates#tab=active~checked%2Citems~checked&title=Hippocrates%20−%20Britannica%20Online%20Encyclopedia. Accessed July 31, 2008.
4. Sarma PJ. Hindu medicine and its antiquity. *Ann Med Hist.* 1931;3:318.
5. Furrow BR, Greaney TL, Johnson SH, et al. *Health Law,* 2nd ed. St. Paul, MN: West Group; 2000.
6. Kohn LT, Corrigan JM, Donaldson MS (eds). Institute of Medicine. *To Err Is Human: Building a Safer Health System.* Washington, DC: National Academies Press, 1999.
7. Institute of Medicine. *Crossing the Quality Chasm: A New Health System for the 21st Century.* Washington, DC: National Academies Press, 2001.

8. Omnibus Budget Reconciliation Act of 1990, Pub. L. No. 101-508, 4401, 104 Stat. 1388-143 (1990).

9. Health Resources and Services Administration, U.S. Department of Health and Human Services. National Practitioner Data Bank Guidebook. http://www.npdb-hipdb.com/pubs/gb/NPDB_Guidebook.pdf. Accessed August 5, 2008.

10. National Practitioner Data Bank for Adverse Information on Physicians and Other Health Care Practitioners. 45 C.F.R. PART 60. http://law.justia.com/us.cfr/title45/45-1.0.1.1.28.html. Accessed July 31, 2008.

11. National Practitioner Data Bank: Healthcare Integrity and Protection Data Bank. Access to Information. http://www.npdb-hipdb.hrsa.gov/npdb.html. Accessed August 6, 2008.

12. Office for Civil Rights—HIPAA. Medical Privacy—National Standards to Protect the Privacy of Personal Health Information. http://www.hhs.gov/ocr/hipaa. Accessed July 31, 2008.

13. Centers for Medicare and Medicaid Services, Department of Health and Human Services. Transactions and Code Sets Regulations. http://www.cms.hhs.gov/TransactionCodeSets Stands/02_TransactionsandCodeSetsRegulations.asp. Accessed July 31, 2008.

14. National Quality Forum. http://www.qualityforum.org. Accessed October 12, 2008.

15. Geier P. Emerging med-mal strategy: "I'm sorry." Early apology concept spreads. *NLJ*. July 24, 2006. http://www.law.com/jsp/article.jsp?id=1153472732197. Accessed July 31, 2008.

16. Gallagher T, Studder D, Levinson W. Disclosing harmful medical errors to patients. *N Engl J Med*. 2007;356:2713–2719.

17. Tanner L. Apology a tool to avoid malpractice suits: Doctors shown financial benefits. *Boston Globe: National News*. November 12, 2004. http://www.boston.com/news/nation/articles/2004/11/12/apology_a_tool_to_avoid_malpractice_suits. Accessed July 31, 2008.

18. Roberts R. The art of apology: When and how to seek forgiveness. *Fam Pract Manag*. 2007;14(7):44–49.

19. Studdert D, Mello M, Gawande A, et al. Disclosure of medical injury to patients: An improbable risk management strategy. *Health Aff*. 2007;26(1):215–226.

20. DeVille KA. *Medical Malpractice in Nineteenth-Century America: Origins and Legacy*. New York: New York University Press; 1990.

21. Mohr JC. The past and future of medical malpractice litigation. *JAMA*. 2000; 284(7):827–829.

22. Agency for Healthcare Research and Quality, U.S. Department of Health and Human Services. Pay-for-Performance: A Decision Guide for Purchasers. http://www.ahrq.gov/qual/p4pguide2.htm. Accessed August 26, 2008.

23. Federal Trade Commission. Antitrust Guidelines for Collaborations among Competitors. Report issued by the Federal Trade Commission and the U.S. Department of Justice. April 2000. http://www.ftc.gov/os/2000/04/ftcdojguidelines.pdf. Accessed October 17, 2008.

24. Medicare Mediation Program. IPRO. http://consumers.ipro.org/index/med-mediation. Accessed August 15, 2008.

25. Expert Pages. Compromise and Offers to Compromise: Federal Rules of Evidence (Article IV)—Relevancy and Its Limits. http://expertpages.com/federal/a4.htm. Accessed August 15, 2008.

26. Beauchamp TL, Childress J. *Principles in Biomedical Ethics*, 5th ed. Oxford/New York: Oxford University Press; 2001.

27. Emanuel EJ, Wendler D, Grady C. What makes clinical research ethical? *JAMA*. 2000; 283(20):2701–2711.

28. Baily MA, Bottrell M, Lynn J, Jennings B. The ethics of using QI methods to improve health care quality and safety. *Hastings Center Report*. 2006;36(4).

29. Palevsky PM, Washington MS, Stevenson JA, et al. Improving compliance with the dialysis prescription as a strategy to increase the delivered dose of hemodialysis: An ESRD Network 4 quality improvement project. *Adv Ren Replace Ther.* 2000;13(1):67–70.

30. U.S. Department of Health and Human Services, the National Commission for the Protection of Human Subjects of Biomedical and Behavioral Research. The Belmont Report. http://www.hhs.gov/ohrp/humansubjects/guidance/belmont.htm. Accessed July 31, 2008.

31. Bellin E, Dubler NN. The quality improvement-research divide and the need for external oversight. *Am J Public Health.* 2001;91(9):1512–1517.

32. National Institute of Health Office of Human Subjects Research. The Nuremberg Code: Regulations and Ethical Guidelines. http://ohsr.od.nih.gov/guidelines/nuremberg.html. Accessed July 31, 2008.

33. The World Medical Association. Ethics Unit: Declaration of Helsinki. http://www.wma.net/e/ethicsunit/helsinki.htm. Accessed July 31, 2008.

34. Centers for Disease Control and Prevention, U.S. Public Health Service. Syphilis Study at Tuskegee. http://www.cdc.gov/tuskegee/timeline.htm. Accessed July 31, 2008.

35. American College of Medical Quality. Professional Policies. http://www.acmq.org/policies/index.cfm. Accessed July 31, 2008.

## Additional Resources–Further Reading

HIPAA: http://www.hhs.gov/ocr/hipaa
National Practitioner Data Bank: http://www.npdb-hipdb.hrsa.gov
National Quality Forum: http://www.qualityforum.org
Sorry Works! Coalition: http://www.sorryworks.net

# Index